EXAMKRACKERS

MCAT

Verbal Reasoning

and

Math

3rd Edition

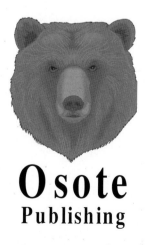

Osote
Publishing

ISBN 1-893858-17-0 (Volume 2)
ISBN 1-893858-20-0 (5 Volume Set)

3rd Edition

To purchase additional copies of this book or the rest of the 5 volume set, call
1-888-572-2536 or fax orders to 1-201-996-1153.

examkrackers.com

osote.com

audioosmosis.com

Inside cover design consultant: Fenwick Design Inc. (212) 246-9722; (201) 944-4337

Printed in Hong Kong

Acknowledgements

Although I am the author, the hard work and expertise of many individuals contributed to this book. The idea of writing in two voices, a science voice and an MCAT voice, was the creative brainchild of my imaginative friend Jordan Zaretsky. I would like to thank Scott Calvin for lending his exceptional pedagogic skills to this project. I also must thank three years worth of EXAMKRACKERS students for doggedly questioning everything in the book. Finally, I wish to thank my wife, Silvia, for her support during the difficult times in the past and those that lie ahead.

Introduction

The following guidelines should be followed when working an MCAT science passage:

1. **Read the passage first.** Regardless of your level of science ability, you should read the passage. Passages often give special conditions that you would have no reason to suspect without reading and which can invalidate an otherwise correct answer.

2. **Read quickly; do not try to master the information given in the passage.** Passages are full of information both useful *and irrelevant* to the adjoining questions. Do not waste time by attempting to gain complete understanding of the passage.

3. **Quickly check tables, graphs, and charts.** Do not spend time studying tables, graphs, and charts. Often, no questions will be asked concerning their content. Instead, quickly check headings, titles, axes, and obvious trends.

4. **When multiple hypotheses or experiments are posited, make note of obvious contrasts in the margin alongside the respective paragraphs.** Making note in the margin will accomplish two things. First, it will distinguish firmly in your mind each of the hypotheses or experiments. (At least one question will require such discernment.) Second, by labeling them you prevent confusion and thus obviate rereading (and avoid wasting precious time).

5. **Pay close attention to detail in the questions.** The key to a question is often found in a single word, such as "*net* force" or "*constant* velocity".

6. **Read answer choices immediately, before doing calculations.** Answer choices give information. Often a question that appears to require extensive calculations can be solved by intuition or estimation due to limited reasonable answer choices. Many answer choices can be eliminated for having the wrong units, being nonsensical, or other reasons.

7. **If time is a factor for you, skip the questions and/or passages that you find difficult.** If you usually do not finish this section, then make sure that you at least answer all of the easy questions. In other words, guess at the difficult questions and come back to them if you have time. **Be sure to make time to answer all of the free-standing questions.** The free-standing questions are usually easier than those based on passages.

MCAT Math

MCAT math will not test your math skills beyond the contents of this chapter. The MCAT <u>does</u> test knowledge of the following up to a second year high school algebra level: ratios; proportions; square roots; exponents and logarithms; scientific notation; quadratic and simultaneous equations; graphs. In addition, the MCAT tests: vector addition, subtraction; basic trigonometry; very basic probabilities. The MCAT <u>does</u> <u>not</u> test dot product, cross product or calculus.

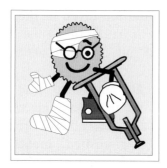

Calculators are neither allowed on the MCAT, nor would they be helpful. From this moment until MCAT day, you should do all math problems in your head whenever possible. Do not use a calculator, and use your pencil as seldom as possible, when you do any math.

This is me after I hurt myself with complicated calculations on my first MCAT.

If you find yourself doing a lot of calculations on the MCAT, it's a good indication that you are doing something wrong. As a rule of thumb, **spend no more than 3 minutes on any MCAT physics question**. Once you have spent 3 minutes on a question with no resolution, you should stop what you're doing and read the question again for a simple answer. If you don't see a simple answer, you should make your best guess and move to the next question.

Rounding

Exact numbers are rarely useful on the MCAT. In order to save time and avoid errors when making calculations on the test, **always use round numbers**. For instance, the gravitational constant **_g_ should always be rounded up to 10 m/s^2** for the purpose of calculations, even when instructed by the MCAT to do otherwise. Calculations like 23.4 x 9.8 should be thought of as "something less than 23.4 x 10, which equals something less than 234 or less than 2.34x10^2." Thus if you see a question requiring the above calculations followed by these answer choices:

    A.   1.24x10^2
    B.   1.81x10^2
    C.   2.28x10^2
    D.   2.35x10^2

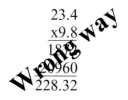

Wrong way

Answer is something less than 23.4 x 10 = 234

Right way

answer choice C is the closest answer under 2.34×10^2, and C should be chosen quickly without resorting to complicated calculations. Rarely will there be two possible answer choices close enough to prevent a correct selection after rounding. If two answer choices on the MCAT are so close that you find you have to write down the math, it's probably because you've made a mistake. If you find yourself in that situation, look again at the question for a simple solution. If you don't see it, guess and go on.

It is helpful to **remain aware of the direction in which you have rounded**. In the above example, since answer choice D is closer to 234 than answer choice C, you may have been tempted to choose it. However, a quick check on the direction in which we rounded would confirm that 9.8 was rounded upward so our answer should be less than 234. Again, assuming the above calculations were necessary to arrive at the answer, an answer choice which would prevent the use of rounding, like 2.32×10^2 for instance, simply would not appear as an answer choice on a real MCAT. It would not appear for the very reason that such an answer choice would force the test taker to spend time making complicated calculations, and those aren't the skills the MCAT is designed to test.

If a series of calculations is used where rounding is performed at each step, the rounding errors can be compounded and the resulting answer can be useless. For instance, we may be required to take the above example and further divide "23.4 x 9.8" by 4.4. We might round 4.4 down to 4, and divide 240 by 4 to get 60; however, each of our roundings would have increased our result compounding the error. Instead, it is better to round 4.4 up to 5, dividing 235 by 5 to get 47. This is closer to the exact answer of 52.1182. In an attempt to increase the accuracy of multiple estimations, **try to compensate for upward rounding with downward rounding in the same calculations**.

Notice, in the example, that when we increase the denominator, we are decreasing the entire term. For instance:

$$\frac{625}{24} = 26.042 \qquad \frac{625}{25} = 25$$

Rounding 24 up to 25 results in a decrease in the overall term.

When rounding squares remember that you are really rounding twice. $(2.2)^2$ is really 2.2 x 2.2, so when we say that the answer is something greater than 4 we need to keep in mind that it is significantly greater because we have rounded down twice. One way to increase your accuracy is to round just one of the 2.2s, leaving you with something greater than 4.4. This is much closer to the exact answer of 4.84.

Another strategy for rounding an exponential term is to remember that difficult-to-solve exponential terms must lie between two easy-to-solve exponential terms. Thus 2.2^2 is between 2^2 and 3^2, closer to 2^2. This strategy is especially helpful for square roots. The square root of 21 must be between the square root of 16 and the square root of 25. Thus, the MCAT square root of 21 must be between 5 and 4 or about 4.6.

$$\sqrt{25} = 5$$
$$\sqrt{21} = ?$$
$$\sqrt{16} = 4$$

For more complicated roots, recall that any root is simply a fractional exponent. For instance, the square root of 9 is the same as $9^{1/2}$. This means that the fourth root of 4 is $4^{1/4}$. This is the same as $(4^{1/2})^{1/2}$ or $\sqrt{2}$. We can combine these techniques to solve even more complicated roots:

$$\sqrt[3]{27} = 3$$
$$4^{2/3} = \sqrt[3]{4^2} = \sqrt[3]{16} = ? = 2.51$$
$$\sqrt[3]{8} = 2$$

It's worth your time to memorize $\sqrt{2} \approx 1.4$ and $\sqrt{3} \approx 1.7$.

The MCAT is likely to give you any values that you need for trigonometric functions; however, since MCAT typically uses common angles, it is a good idea to be very familiar with trigonometric values for common angles. Use the paradigm below to remember the values of common angles. Notice that the sine values are the reverse of the cosine values. Also notice that the numbers under the radical are 0, 1, 2, 3 and 4 from top to bottom for the sine function and bottom to top for the cosine function, and all are divided by 2.

θ	sine	cosine
$0°$	$\dfrac{\sqrt{0}}{2}$	$\dfrac{\sqrt{4}}{2}$
$30°$	$\dfrac{\sqrt{1}}{2}$	$\dfrac{\sqrt{3}}{2}$
$45°$	$\dfrac{\sqrt{2}}{2}$	$\dfrac{\sqrt{2}}{2}$
$60°$	$\dfrac{\sqrt{3}}{2}$	$\dfrac{\sqrt{1}}{2}$
$90°$	$\dfrac{\sqrt{4}}{2}$	$\dfrac{\sqrt{0}}{2}$

Less practiced test takers may perceive a rounding strategy as risky. On the contrary, **the test makers actually design their answers with a rounding strategy in mind**. Complicated numbers can be intimidating to anyone not comfortable with a rounding strategy.

Questions:

Solve the following problems by rounding.
Do not use a pencil or a calculator.

1.

$$\frac{5.4 \times 7.1 \times 3.2}{4.6^2}$$

A. 2.2
B. 3.8
C. 5.8
D. 7.9

2.

$$\frac{\sqrt{360 \times 9.8}}{6.2}$$

A. 9.6
B. 13.2
C. 17.3
D. 20.2

3.

$$\frac{(\sqrt{2}) \times 23}{50}$$

A. 0.12
B. 0.49
C. 0.65
D. 1.1

4.

$$\frac{(2 \times 45)^2}{9.8 \times 21}$$

A. 11
B. 39
C. 86
D. 450

5.

$$\sqrt{\frac{2 \times 9.8^2}{49}}$$

A. 0.3
B. 0.8
C. 1.2
D. 2

Answers:

1. C is correct. The exact answer is 5.7981.
2. A is correct. The exact answer is 9.5802.
3. C is correct. The exact answer is 0.65054.
4. B is correct. The exact answer is 39.359.
5. D is correct. The exact answer is 1.9799.

Scientific Notation

One important math skill tested rigorously by the MCAT is your ability to use scientific notation. In order to maximize your MCAT score, you must be familiar with the techniques and shortcuts of scientific notation. Although it may not seem so, scientific notation was designed to make math easier, and it does. You should practice the following techniques until you come to view scientific notation as a valuable ally.

This manual will define the terms in scientific notation as follows:

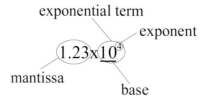

Magnitude: You should try to gain a feel for the exponential aspect of scientific notation. 10^{-8} is much greater than 10^{-12}. It is 10,000 times greater! Thus, when comparing one solution whose concentration of particles is 3.2×10^{-11} mol/L with a second solution whose concentration of particles is 4.1×10^{-9} mol/L, you should visualize the second solution as hundreds of times more concentrated than the first. Pay special attention to magnitudes when adding. For example try solving:

$$3.74 \times 10^{-15}$$
$$+ \underline{6.43 \times 10^{-3}}$$

On the MCAT, the answer is simply 6.43×10^{-3}. This is true because 6.43×10^{-3} is so much greater than 3.74×10^{-15} that 3.74×10^{-15} is negligible. Thus you can round off the answer to 6.43×10^{-3}. After all, the exact answer is 0.00643000000000374. Try solving:

$$5.32 \times 10^{-4}$$
$$\times \underline{1.12 \times 10^{-13}}$$

The MCAT answer is something greater than 5.3×10^{-17}. We cannot ignore the smaller number in this case because we are multiplying. **In addition or subtraction, a number 100 times or more smaller can be considered negligible. This is not true in multiplication or division**.

The fastest way to add or subtract numbers in scientific notation is to make the exponents match. For instance:

$$2.76 \times 10^4$$
$$+\underline{6.91 \times 10^5}$$

The MCAT answer is something less than 7.2×10^5. To get this answer quickly we match the exponents and rewrite the equation as follows:

$$2.76 \times 10^4$$
$$+\underline{69.1 \times 10^4}$$

This is similar to the algebraic equation:

$$2.76y$$
$$+\underline{69.1y}$$

where y equals 10^4. We simply add the coefficients of y. Rounding, we have $3y + 69y = 72y$. Thus 72×10^4, or 7.2×10^5 is the answer.

When rearranging 6.91×10^5 to 69.1×10^4, we simply multiply by 10/10 (a form of 1). In other words, we divide 72 by 10 and multiply 10^4 by 10.

$$\begin{array}{c} \times 10 \\ 6.91 \times 10^5 = 69.1 \times 10^4 \\ \div 10 \end{array}$$

A useful mnemonic for remembering which way to move the decimal point when we add or subtract from the exponent is to use the acronym LARS,

Left **A**dd, **R**ight **S**ubtract

Multiplication and division:

When multiplying similar bases with exponents add the exponents; when dividing, subtract the exponents. $10^4 \times 10^5 = 10^9$. $10^4 / 10^{-6} = 10^{10}$.

When multiplying or dividing with scientific notation, we deal with the exponential terms and mantissa separately, *regardless of the number of terms*. For instance:

$$\frac{(3.2 \times 10^4) \times (4.9 \times 10^{-8})}{(2.8 \times 10^{-7})}$$

should be rearranged to:

$$\frac{3 \times 5}{3} \times \frac{10^4 \times 10^{-8}}{10^{-7}}$$

giving us an MCAT answer of something greater than 5×10^3. (The exact answer, 5.6×10^3, is greater than our estimate because we decreased one term in the numerator by more than we increased the other, which would result in a low estimate, and because we increased the term in the denominator, which also results in a low estimate.)

When taking a term written in scientific notation to some power (such as squaring or cubing it), we also deal with the decimal and exponent separately. The MCAT answer to:

$$(3.1 \times 10^7)^2$$

is something greater than 9×10^{14}. Recall that when taking an exponential term to a power, we multiply the exponents.

The first step in taking the square root of a term in scientific notation is to make the exponent even. Then we take the square root of the mantissa and exponential term separately.

$$\sqrt{8.1 \times 10^5}$$

Make the exponent even.

$$\sqrt{81 \times 10^4}$$

Take the square root of the mantissa and exponential term separately.

$$\sqrt{81} \times \sqrt{10^4} = 9 \times 10^2$$

Notice how much efficient this method is. What is the square root of 49,000? Most students start thinking about 700, or 70, or something with a 7 in it. By using the scientific notation method, we quickly see that there is no 7 involved at all.

$$\sqrt{49,000} = \sqrt{4.9 \times 10^4} = 2.1 \times 10^2$$

Try finding the square root of 300 and the square root of 200.

Questions:

Solve the following problems without a calculator. Try not to use a pencil.

1.
$$\frac{2.3 \times 10^7 \times 5.2 \times 10^{-5}}{4.3 \times 10^2}$$

A. 1.2×10^{-1}
B. 2.8
C. 3.1×10
D. 5.6×10^2

2.
$$(2.5 \times 10^{-7} \times 3.7 \times 10^{-6}) + 4.2 \times 10^2$$

A. 1.3×10^{-11}
B. 5.1×10^{-10}
C. 4.2×10^2
D. 1.3×10^{15}

3.
$$(1.1 \times 10^{-4} + 8.9 \times 10^{-5})^{\frac{1}{2}}$$

A. 1.1×10^{-2}
B. 1.4×10^{-2}
C. 1.8×10^{-2}
D. 2.0×10^{-2}

4.
$$\frac{1}{2} (3.4 \times 10^2) (2.9 \times 10^8)^2$$

A. 1.5×10^{18}
B. 3.1×10^{18}
C. 1.4×10^{19}
D. 3.1×10^{19}

5.
$$\frac{1.6 \times 10^{-19} \times 15}{36^2}$$

A. 1.9×10^{-21}
B. 2.3×10^{-17}
C. 1.2×10^{-9}
D. 3.2×10^{-9}

Answers:

1. B is correct. The exact answer is 2.7814
2. C is correct. The other numbers are insignificant
3. B is correct. The exact answer is 1.4107×10^{-2}
4. C is correct. The exact answer is 1.4297×10^{19}
5. A is correct. The exact answer is 1.8519×10^{-19}

Proportions

On the MCAT, proportional relationships between variables can often be used to circumvent lengthy calculations or, in some cases, the MCAT question simply asks the test taker to identify the relationship directly. When the MCAT asks for the change in one variable due to the change in another, they are making the assumption that all other variables remain constant.

In the equation $F = ma$, we see that if we double F while holding m constant, a doubles. If we triple F, a triples. The same relationship holds for m and F. This type of relationship is called a **direct proportion**.

$$\overset{2}{F} = m\overset{2}{a}$$

F and a are directly proportional.

Notice that if we change the equation to $F = ma + b$, the directly proportional relationships are destroyed. Now if we double F while holding all variables besides a constant, a increases, but does not double. **In order for variables to be directly proportional to each other, they must both be in the numerator or denominator when they are on opposite sides of the equation, or one must be in the numerator while the other is in the denominator when they are on the same side of the equation. In addition, all sums or differences in the equation must be contained in parentheses and multiplied by the rest of the equation. No variables within the sums or differences will be directly proportional to any other variable.**

If we examine the relationship between m and a, in $F = ma$, we see that when F is held constant and m is doubled, a is reduced by a factor of 2. This type of relationship is called **inversely proportional**. Again the relationship is destroyed if we add b to the equation. **In order for variables to be inversely proportional to each other, they must both be in the numerator or denominator when they are on the same side of the equation, or one must be in the numerator while the other is in the denominator when they are on opposite sides of the equation. In addition, all sums or differences in the equation must be contained in parentheses and multiplied by the rest of the equation. No variables within the sums or differences will be directly proportional to any other variable.**

$$F = \underset{2}{m}\overset{2}{a}$$

m and a are inversely proportional.

If we examine a more complicated equation, the same rules apply. However, we have to take care when dealing with exponents. One method to solve an equation using proportions is as follows. Suppose we are given the following equation:

$$Q = \frac{\Delta P \pi r^4}{8 \eta L}$$

This is Poiseuille's Law. The volume flow rate Q of a real fluid through a horizontal pipe is equal to the product of the change in pressure ΔP, π, and the radius of the pipe to the fourth power r^4, divided by 8 times the viscosity η and the length L of the pipe.

Water ($\eta = 1.80 \times 10^{-3}$ Pa s) flows through a pipe with a 14.0 cm radius at 2.00 L/s. An engineer wishes to increase the length of the pipe from 10.0 m to 40.0 m without changing the flow rate or the pressure difference. What radius must the pipe have?

    A. 12.1 cm
    B. 14.0 cm
    C. 19.8 cm
    D. 28.0 cm

Answer: The only way to answer this question is with proportions. Most of the information is given to distract you. Notice that the difference in pressure between the ends of the pipe is not even given and the flow rate would have to be converted to m^3/s. To answer this question using proportions, multiply L by 4 and r by x. Now pull out the 4 and the x. We know from that, by definition, $Q = \Delta P \pi r^4 / 8 \eta L$; thus, $x^4/4$ must equal 1. Solve for x, and this is the change in the radius. The radius must be increased by a factor of about 1.4. 14 x 1.4 = 19.6. The new radius is approximately19.6 cm. The closest answer is **C**.

$$Q = \frac{\Delta P \pi r^4}{8 \eta L}$$

$$Q = \frac{\Delta P \pi (xr)^4}{8 \eta (4L)}$$

$$Q = \frac{\Delta P \pi r^4}{8 \eta L} \cdot \frac{x^4}{4}$$

$$4 = x^4$$

$$x = \sqrt{2}$$

Questions:

1. The coefficient of surface tension is given by the equation $\gamma = (F - mg)/(2L)$, where F is the net force necessary to pull a submerged wire of weight mg and length L through the surface of the fluid in question. The force required to remove a submerged wire from water was measured and recorded. If an equal force is required to remove a separate submerged wire with the same mass but twice the length from fluid x, what is the coefficient of surface tension for fluid x. ($\gamma_{water} = 0.073$ mN/m)

   A. 0.018 mN/m
   B. 0.037 mN/m
   C. 0.073 mN/m
   D. 0.146 mN/m

2. A solid sphere rotating about a central axis has a moment of inertia $I = {}^2/_5 MR^2$ where R is the radius of the sphere and M is its mass. Although Callisto, a moon of Jupiter, is approximately the same size as the planet Mercury, Mercury is 3 times as dense. How do their moments of inertia compare?

   A. The moment of inertia for Mercury is 9 times greater than for Callisto.
   B. The moment of inertia for Mercury is 3 times greater than for Callisto.
   C. The moment of inertia for Mercury is equal to the moment of inertia for Callisto.
   D. The moment of inertia for Callisto is 3 times greater than for Mercury.

3. The force of gravity on an any object due to earth is given by the equation $F = G(m_o M/r^2)$ where G is the gravitational constant, M is the mass of the earth, m_o is the mass of the object and r is the distance between the center of mass of the earth and the center of mass of the object. If a rocket weighs 3.6×10^6 N at the surface of the earth what is the force on the rocket due to gravity when the rocket has reached an altitude of 1.2×10^4 km? ($G = 6.67 \times 10^{-11}$ Nm²/kg², radius of the earth $= 6370$ km, mass of the earth $= 5.98 \times 10^{24}$ kg)

   A. 1.2×10^5 N
   B. 4.3×10^5 N
   C. 4.8×10^6 N
   D. 9.6×10^6 N

4. The kinetic energy E of an object is given by $E = \frac{1}{2} mv^2$ where m is the object's mass and v is the velocity of the object. If the velocity of an object decreases by a factor of 2 what will happen its kinetic energy?

   A. Kinetic energy will increase by a factor of 2.
   B. Kinetic energy will increase by a factor of 4.
   C. Kinetic energy will decrease by a factor of 2.
   D. Kinetic energy will decrease by a factor of 4.

5. Elastic potential energy in a spring is directly proportional to the square of the displacement of one end of the spring from its rest position while the other end remains fixed. If the elastic potential energy in the spring is 100 J when it is compressed to half its rest length, what is its energy when it is compressed to one fourth its rest length.

    A. 50 J
    B. 150 J
    C. 200 J
    D. 225 J

Answers:

1. B is correct. γ and L are inversely proportional.

    $$\frac{F-mg}{2\cancel{L}^2} = \cancel{\gamma}_2$$

2. B is correct. Since the bodies are the same size and Mercury is 3 times more dense, Mercury is 3 times more massive. Mass is directly proportional to moment of inertia.
3. B is correct. If you are good with scientific notation, it is easy to see that r is tripled. Since the square of r inversely proportional to F, F must be divided by 9.
4. D is correct. E is directly proportional to v^2.
5. D is correct. If we imagine a spring 100 cm long at rest (We can use any spring length but 100 is always a good choice.) then the initial displacement is 50 cm and the final displacement is 75 cm. The displacement is increased by a factor of 1.5 thus the energy is increased by a factor of 1.5^2. 1.5^2 is greater than 1.4^2 or greater than 2. Thus the energy is greater than 2 x 100.

Graphs

The MCAT requires that you recognize the graphical relationship between two variables in certain types of equations. The three graphs below are the most commonly used. You should memorize them. The first is a directly proportional relationship; the second is an exponential relationship; and the third is an inversely proportional relationship.

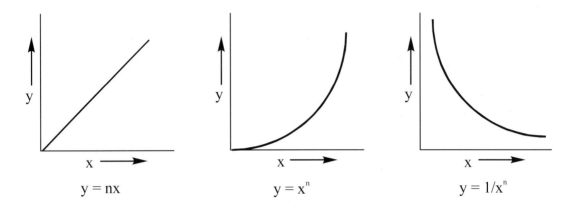

$$y = nx \qquad\qquad y = x^n \qquad\qquad y = 1/x^n$$

(Note: n is greater zero for the $y = nx$, and n is greater than one for the other two graphs.) Notice that, if we add a constant b to the right side, the graph is simply raised vertically by an amount b.

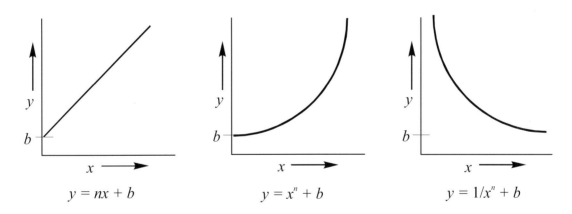

$$y = nx + b \qquad\qquad y = x^n + b \qquad\qquad y = 1/x^n + b$$

As long as the value of n is within the given parameters, the general shape of the graph will not change. When graphs are unitless, multiplying the right side of an equation by a positive constant will not change the shape of the graph. If one side of the equation is negative, or multiplied by a negative constant, the graph is reflected across the x axis.

Whenever the MCAT asks you to identify the graphical relationship between two variables you should assume that all other variables in the equations are constants unless told otherwise. Next, manipulate the equation into one of the above forms (with or without the added constant b, and choose the corresponding graph.

If you are unsure of a graphical relationship, plug in 1 for all variables except the variables in the question and then plug in 0, 1, and 2 for x and solve for y. Plot your results and look for the general corresponding shape.

Questions:

1. The height of an object dropped from a building in the absence of air resistance is given by the equation $h = h_o + v_ot + \frac{1}{2} gt^2$, where h_o and v_o are the initial height and velocity respectively and g is -10 m/s^2. If v_o is zero which graph best represents the relationship between h and t?

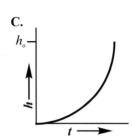

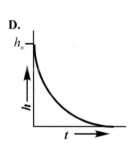

2. Which of the following graphs best describes the magnitude of the force (F) on a spring obeying Hooke's law ($F = -k\Delta x$) as it is compressed to Δx_{max}.

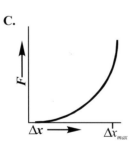

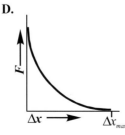

3. Which of the following graphs shows the relationship between frequency and wavelength of electromagnetic radiation through a vacuum. ($c = v\lambda$)

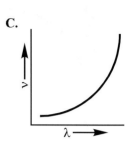

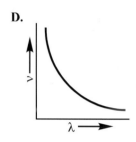

4. Which of the following graphs best describes the magnitude of the electrostatic force $F = k(qq)/r^2$ created by an object with negative charge on an object with a positive charge as the distance r between them changes.

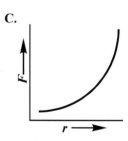

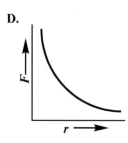

5. Which of the following graphs demonstrates the relationship between power P and work W done by a machine. ($P = W/t$)

A.

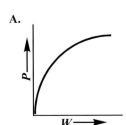

C.

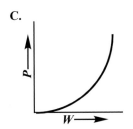

B.

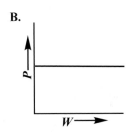

D.

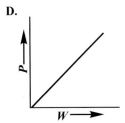

Answers:

1. A is correct. Since v_o is zero we have $h = h_o + \frac{1}{2} gt^2$. Since g is in the opposite direction to h, and h_o is a constant we can rewrite this equation as $h = -\frac{1}{2} gt^2 + h_o$ where $g = 10$. This is the same form as $y = x^n$. The negative sign flips the graph vertically. In addition a constant has been added to the right side so the graph intercepts the y axis at h_o.
2. A is correct. The question asks for magnitude. Thus the negative sign is ignored and the equation has the form $y = nx$.
3. D is correct. Manipulation of this formula produces $v = c/\lambda$. Which is in the form of $y = 1/x$.
4. D is correct. The form of this equation is $y = 1/x^n$. The negative can be ignored because the question asks for magnitude.
5. D is correct. The equation has the form $y = nx$ where n is $1/t$.

Verbal Lecture 1: Strategy and Tactics

The Layout of the Verbal Reasoning Section

The verbal reasoning section of the MCAT is composed of nine passages, averaging 600 words per passage. Generally, a passage discusses an area from the humanities, social sciences, or natural sciences. Six to ten multiple-choice questions follow each passage for a total of **65 questions**. Answers to these questions do not require information beyond the text of the passage. The test taker has **85 minutes** to complete the entire section.

Others Verbal Strategies

Dogma about the verbal section is abundant and free, and that's an accurate reflection of its value. There are many cock-a-mamie verbal strategies touted by various prep companies, academics and well-wishers. **We strongly suggest that you ignore them.** Most are designed to be marketable (to make money) as opposed to being efficient (raise your score). Desperate techniques such as mapping and skimming are prime examples. Some colleges offer classes designed specifically to improve reading comprehension in the MCAT verbal section. Typically, such classes resemble English 101. They are taught by humanities professors who have never even seen a real MCAT verbal section. Being a humanities professor does not qualify you as an expert at the MCAT verbal section. Predictably, the success rate of these classes is very poor. There are those who will tell you that a strong performance on the verbal section requires speed-reading techniques. This is not true. Most speed-reading techniques actually prove to be an impediment to score improvements by shifting focus from understanding to technique. As you will soon see, speed is not the key to a good MCAT verbal score. Please abandon all your preconceived notions concerning the MCAT verbal section.

Take Our Advice

Most smart students listen to advice, then pick and choose the suggestions that they find reasonable while disregarding the rest. This is not the most efficient approach for preparing to take the MCAT verbal section. Please abandon all your old ideas about verbal and **follow our advice to the letter**.

Expected improvement

Taking the MCAT verbal section is an art. (Not exactly what a science major wants to hear.) Like any art form, improvement comes gradually with lots of practice. Imagine attending a class in portraiture taught by a great artist. You wouldn't expect to become a Raphael after your first lesson, but you would expect to improve after weeks of coaching. The verbal section is the same way. Follow our directions to the letter, and you will see dramatic improvements over time.

The EXAMKRACKERS Approach to MCAT Verbal Reasoning

We shall examine the verbal section on two levels: strategic and tactical. The strategic point of view will encompass the general approach to the section as a whole. The tactical point of view will break the section down, passage by passage, and question by question.

Strategy

There are four aspects to strategy:

1. **Energy**
2. **Focus**
3. **Confidence**
4. **Timing**

Energy

Pull your chair close to the table. Sit up straight. Place your feet flat on the floor, and be alert. This may seem to be obvious advice to some, but it is rarely followed. Test-takers often look for the most comfortable position to read the passage. Do you really believe that you do your best thinking when you're relaxed? Webster's Dictionary gives the definition of relaxed as "freed from or lacking in precision or stringency." Your cerebral cortex is most active when your sympathetic nervous system is in high gear, so don't deactivate it by relaxing. Your posture makes a big difference to your score.

One strategy of the test writers is to wear you down with the verbal section before you begin the science sections. You must mentally prepare yourself for the tremendous amount of energy necessary for a strong performance on the verbal section. Like an intellectual athlete, you must train yourself to concentrate for long periods of time. You must improve your reading comprehension stamina. **Practice! Practice! Practice!** And **always give 100% effort when you practice**. If you give less than 100% when you practice, you will be teaching yourself to relax when you take the verbal, and you will be lowering your score. It is more productive to watch TV than to practice with less than complete effort. If you are not mentally worn after finishing three or more verbal passages, then you have not tried hard enough, and you have trained yourself to do it incorrectly. Even when you are only practicing, sit up straight in your chair and attack each passage.

Focus

The verbal section is made up of nine passages with both interesting and boring topics. It is sometimes difficult to switch gears from "the migration patterns of the Alaskan tit-mouse" to "economic theories of the post-Soviet Union." In other words, sometimes you may be reading one passage while thinking about the prior passage. You must learn to **focus your attention on the task at hand.** We will discuss methods to increase your focus when we discuss tactics.

During the real MCAT, it is not unlikely that unexpected interruptions occur. People get physically ill, nervous students breath heavily, air conditioners break down, and lights go out. Your score will not be adjusted for unwelcome interruptions, and excuses will not get you into med school, so learn to focus and **ignore distractions**.

Confidence

There are two aspects to confidence on the verbal section: 1) **be confident of your score** and 2) **be arrogant when you read**.

Imagine taking a multiple choice exam and narrowing 50% of the questions down to just two answer choices, and then guessing. On a physics exam, this would almost certainly indicate a very low grade. Yet, this exact situation describes a stellar performance on the verbal section of the MCAT. Everyone of whom we know that has earned a perfect score on the verbal section (including many of our own students), has guessed on a large portion of the answers. The test writers are aware that most students can predict their grade on science exams based upon their performance, and that guessing makes science majors extremely uncomfortable. The verbal section is the most dissatisfying in terms of perceived performance. You should realize that even the best test takers finish the verbal section with some frustration and insecurity concerning their performance. A perceived dissatisfactory performance early in the testing day is likely to reflect poorly in scores on the science sections. You should assume that you have guessed correctly on every answer of the verbal section and get psyched to ace the science sections.

The second aspect of confidence concerns how you read the passage. Read the passages as if you were a Harvard professor grading high school essays. Read critically. If you are confused while reading the passage, assume that it is the passage writer, and not you, who is at fault. If you find a contradiction in the reasoning of the argument, trust your reasoning ability that you are correct. The questions will focus on the author's argument and you must be confident of the strong and weak points. In order to identify the strong and weak points, you must read with confidence.

Timing

If you want a 10 or better on the verbal section, you must read every passage and attempt to answer every question. If you want to go to medical school, you should attempt to score 10 on the verbal section. Therefore, **read every passage in the order given, and attempt every question**.

Skipping around in the verbal section to find the easiest passages is a marketable strategy but an obvious waste of time. It is a bad idea that makes a lot of money for some prep companies because it's an easy trick to sell. 'Cherry picking' is an unfortunate carry over from SAT strategy where it works because the questions are prearranged in order of difficulty. On the MCAT, some passages are difficult to read, but have easy questions; some passages are easy to read, but have difficult questions. Some passages start out difficult and finish easy. You have no way of knowing if a passage is easy or difficult until you have read the entire passage and attempted all the questions.

If you begin reading a passage and are asking yourself "Shall I continue, or shall I move on to the next passage? Is this passage easy or difficult?", then you are not reading with confidence, you are not concentrating on what the author is saying, and you are wasting valuable time. Your energy and focus should be on doing well on each passage, not on trying to decide which passage to do first.

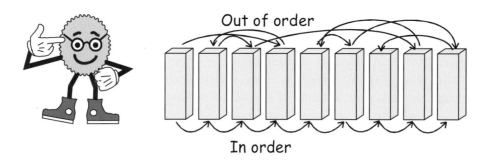

Let's see. I must knock down all nine blocks. Is it faster and more efficient to knock them down in order or out of order?

Check your timer only once during the verbal section. Constantly checking your timer is distracting and not very useful since some passages take longer to finish than others. Instead, **check your timer only once, and after you have finished the fifth passage.** You should have about 40 minutes left. A well-practiced test taker will develop a sense of timing acute enough to obviate looking at a timer at all.

Don't spend too much time with the difficult questions. **Guess at the difficult questions and move on**. Guessing is very difficult for good students, who are accustomed to being certain of the answer. Test writers are aware of this, and use it to their advantage. Learn to give up on difficult questions so that you have more time on easier questions. Giving up on difficult questions is one of the keys to finishing the exam.

Many test-takers are able to guess on difficult questions during a practice exam, but when it comes to the real MCAT, they want to be certain of the answers. This meticulous approach has cost such students as many as 3 points on their scaled score. Learn to let go of difficult questions.

Finish the entire section with two minutes to spare, no more, no less. If you have more than two minutes to spare, you missed questions on which you could have spent more time. Finishing the exam early and returning to difficult questions is not a good strategy. The stress of exam taking actually makes you more perspicacious while you take the exam. When you finish an exam, even if you intend to go back and check your work, you typically breath a sigh of relief. Upon doing so, you lose your perspicacity. The best strategy is to use your time efficiently during your first and only pass through the exam.

Tactics

Although, at first glance, it may not appear so, the following techniques are designed to increase your pace and efficiency. Follow these steps for each passage.

1. **Take a five second break**
2. **Read every word**
3. **Construct a main idea**.
4. **Use all four tools to answer the questions:**

    Tools:
    1) **going back;**
    2) **the main idea;**
    3) **the question stems; and**
    4) **the answer choices.**

The Five Second Break

If you were to observe a room full of MCAT takers just after the sentence "You may break the seal on your test booklet and begin," you would see a room full of people frantically tear open their test booklets, read for 20 to 30 seconds, pause, and then begin rereading from the beginning. Why? Because as they race through the first passage, they are thinking about what is happening to them ("I'm taking the real MCAT! Oh my God!"), and not thinking about what they are reading. They need a moment to become accustomed to the idea that the MCAT has actually begun. They need a moment to focus. However, they don't need 20 to 30 seconds! They take so much time, because they are trying to do two things at once, focus and read, and end up accomplishing neither. This loss of concentration may also occur at the beginning of each new passage, when the test-taker may still be struggling with thoughts of the previous passage while reading the new passage.

If you continued to observe the test-takers, you would see them in the midst of a passage suddenly stop everything, lift up their head, stretch, yawn, or crack their knuckles. This is their beleaguered mind, forcing them to take a break. No one has an attention span 85 minutes long. If you don't allow yourself a break, your mind will take one. How many times have you been reading a passage when suddenly you realize, you weren't concentrating? You're forced to start the passage over. More time is wasted.

There is a simple method to prevent all this lost time. Instead of taking breaks at random, inconvenient moments, plan your breaks. **Before each passage, including the first, take five seconds to focus your thoughts.** Remind yourself to forget the last passage and all other thoughts not related to the task at hand. Remind yourself to sit up straight, concentrate and focus. For these five seconds, look away from the page, stretch your muscles and prepare to give your full attention to the next passage. Then begin and don't break your concentration until you have finished answering all the questions to that passage. The five second break is like a little pep-talk before each passage.

Unfortunately, most students will not take the five second break. Understand one thing. All students will take breaks during the verbal section. Most will take them without realizing it, and most will take them at inopportune moments. If your goal is to get the highest verbal score of which you are capable, you should take the five second break at planned intervals.

Reading the Passage

Most test takers have difficulty finishing the verbal section in the 85 minutes allowed. Many finish as few as six passages. Strangely enough, any premed without a reading disorder is capable of reading 5400 words and taking a one hour nap in 85 minutes. A very slow reader can easily read every word of a 600 word passage in 2 minutes and 30 seconds. Try it! It's true! This leaves over an hour to answer the questions, or 6 minutes and 57 seconds per question set. So why do so many test-takers fail to finish the verbal section? The answer is "because they spend too much time hunting for the answer in the passage, and end up reading the passage many times over." We'll talk more about "going back" to the passage when we discuss where to find the answer choice. For now, just believe us that **you can read every word in the verbal section and easily finish the exam**, so you should.

The people that write the MCAT know that most of us are scientists. They know that we like to find the exact answer to things. Give us a mysterious powder and let us analyze it and we will tell you exactly what it is. Show us the exact words in a passage as an answer choice and we will probably choose it. Don't fall for this trap. The Verbal Section tests your ability to detect and understand ambiguities and gray areas, not details. Rely heavily on your main idea and give little weight to details. If you are highly certain of all your answers on the Verbal Section, then you probably have fallen for all its traps. **Mastering this section is as much an art as a science**. With practice, you will develop a 'feel' for a good MCAT answer. Learn to use this 'feel' to help you move faster through the Verbal Section. If you teach yourself not to expect the concrete certainty that you get with science questions, you will become more comfortable with the Verbal Section and your score will increase.

The biggest mistake you can make on the verbal section is to consciously attempt to remember what you are reading. The vast majority of the questions will not concern the details of the passage and will not be answerable by searching the passage for facts. Most questions are about the main idea of the passage. The main idea will not be found in a list of details. In order to learn the main idea, the passage as a whole must be understood. Read the passage the way you would read an interesting novel; **concentrate on the main idea, not the detail.**

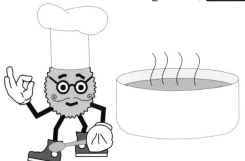

When I create a great soup, you do not taste the salt, and each spice separately. You must experience the whole soup as a single, wonderful *consomme'*. Otherwise you are nothing but a tasteless peasant, and I will not invite you to dinner.

An often posited tactic is to read the questions first; don't do it! You will not remember even one question while you read the passage, much less the 6 to 10 questions that accompany every passage. In fact, a short term memory can contain 5 items; that's why the passages are followed by six or more questions. Not only that, reading the questions first will force you to read for detail and you will never learn the main idea. You will probably end up rereading the passage many times but never straight through. This results in a tremendous waste of time.

Don't circle or underline words. This is another marketing technique that has sold well but is counterproductive. It is very unlikely that underlining or circling a sentence or a word will assist you in answering any questions. Have you ever answered a question correctly because you underlined or circled something in the passage? Underlining and circling words forces you to concentrate on detail; great for the SAT, not good for the MCAT. When you underline or circle something, you are reading it twice. This interrupts the flow of the passage. It distracts you from the main idea. This is an old SAT trick, inappropriately applied to MCAT.

Some of the Verbal topics will fascinate you and some will bore you. The challenge will be to forget the ones that fascinate you as soon as you move to the next passage, and to pay close attention to the ones that bore you as you read them. **Train yourself to become excited and interested in any and every passage topic.** This will increase your comprehension. However, don't become so engrossed in a passage that you slow your pace.

Don't use fancy speed reading techniques where you search for meaningful words or try to read entire phrases in one thought. This will only distract you from your goal. Your reading speed is unlikely to change significantly in 10 weeks, and your reading speed is not the problem anyway. Finishing the entire section depends upon how long you spend on the questions, not how long it takes you to read the passage. You also cannot assume that the passages are written well enough, so that you can read just the first and last sentence of each paragraph. They are often barely intelligible when you read every word. You must read every word, read quickly and concentrate.

Read each passage like you are listening to a friend tell you a very interesting story. Allow the details (names, dates, times) to slip in one ear and out the other, while you wait with baited breath for the main point. The funny thing about this type of reading is that, when you practice it, you can't help but remember most of the details. Even if you were to forget some of the details, it only takes about *5* seconds to find a name, number, or key word in a 600 word passage. Thus, when you run into a rare question about a detail that you've forgotten, it is easy to find the answer. Another convenient aspect of this type of reading is that you are trying to accomplish exactly what the verbal section will be testing: your ability to pick out the main idea. The best thing about this type of reading is that you have practiced it every day of your life. This is the way that you read novels, newspapers and magazines. **Read the passages the way that you read best; read for the main idea.**

When you read, ask yourself "What is the author trying to say? What is his point? Is he in favor of idea A or against it? If this author were sitting right in front of me, would he want to discuss idea A or is his real interest in idea B?" **Create an image of the author in your mind.** Stereotype the author, and then make careful mental note of anything the author says that may not fit that stereotype. Use the stereotype to help guide your intuition on the questions.

The Main Idea

When you have finished reading a passage, take thirty seconds and construct a main idea in the form of one or two complete sentences. Verbal Reasoning Lecture 3 will cover how to construct a main idea. On a timed MCAT, writing the main idea requires too much time, so you should **spend 20 seconds mentally contemplating the main idea before you begin the questions.** After you have completed the entire exam, it is a good idea to go back to each passage and write the main idea for practice.

Answering the Questions

Answering the questions will be covered thoroughly in Verbal Reasoning Lecture 2. For now, attempt to answer the questions based upon the main idea and not the details.

Lecture 2: Answering the Questions

You have four tools to help you find the answer to a question on the verbal section:

1) **going back;**
2) **the main idea;**
3) **the question stems; and**
4) **the answer choices.**

Going Back

'Going back' refers to actually rereading parts of the passage to search for an answer. 'Going back' should be **used only when**:

you know what you're looking for,

and

you know where you can find it.

'Going back' is the most time consuming and least useful of the four tools. Unfortunately, it is the tool most often relied upon by inexperienced test takers. It is true that forgotten details can be found by rereading parts of the passage. However, most questions require an understanding of the main idea, not your memory of details. The main idea cannot be found by rereading parts of the passage.

'Word-for-word' and other traps have been set for the unwary test taker looking for the 'feel-good' answer. The 'feel-good' answer is an answer where a section of the passage seems to unequivocally answer the question so that the test taker *feels good* when choosing it. This is often a trap. Remember, the Verbal Section is ambiguous and a simple clear answer is rarely the correct answer.

You should learn to use 'going back' as seldom as possible. Most of the time you should force yourself to choose the best answer without going back to the passage. This is a difficult lesson to accept, but it is extremely important to achieving your top score. Going back to the passage for anything but a detail will take large amounts of your testing time, and allow the test writers to skew your concept of the main idea by directing you toward specific parts of the passage. **<u>If you are unable to finish the test in the time given, it is because you are overusing the 'going back' tool.</u>**

Questions sometimes refer to line numbers in the passage. **Don't assume that you must go back to the given line number.** Usually these types of questions should be answered without going back to the given line numbers. Often times the most helpful part of the passage in answering the question is nowhere near the lines mentioned. If you do go back, you may have to begin reading 5 lines above the actual reference in order to place the reference in the correct context.

Your number one goal should be to finish the Verbal section. Difficult questions are worth no more than easy questions. **Don't sacrifice five easy questions by spending a long time answering a single difficult question. If you usually finish the Verbal section with time to spare, you can 'go back' to the passage more often; if you don't usually finish the Verbal section, you should reduce the time you spend 'going back' to the passage.**

Main Idea

The main idea is the most powerful tool for answering MCAT verbal questions. We will discuss the main idea in Verbal Reasoning Lecture 3.

Question Stems

**The section that follows includes material from the MCAT Practice Test 1/Practice Items. These materials are reprinted with permission of the Association of American Medical Colleges (AAMC).

The **question stems hold as much information as the passage**. Read them and see how much you can learn about the passage from just the question stems.

1. The author of the passage believes that the fiction written by the current generation of authors:
2. The overall point made by the passage's comparison of movies to fiction is that:
3. According to the passage, John Gardner concedes that preliminary good advice to a beginning writer might be, "Write as if you were a movie camera." The word *concedes* here suggests that:
4. The fact that the author rereads *Under the Volcano* because it has been made into a movie is ironic because it:
5. The passage suggests that a reader who is not bored by a line-by-line description of a room most likely:
6. The passage suggests that if a contemporary writer were to write a novel of great forcefulness, this novel would most likely:
7. The passage places the blame for contemporary writers' loss of readers on the:

Answer the following questions using just the question stems.

1. Based on the question stems, if the author were sitting in front of you, he would probably be most interested in discussing:

    A. popular movies.
    B. movie cameras.
    C. contemporary fiction.
    D. modern reading habits.

2. Based on the question stems, this passage was most likely about:

    A. the impact of modern movies on fiction.
    B. how to write good fiction.
    C. *Under the Volcano*, the book vs. the movie.
    D. how good books often make for bad movies.

The answers are below. Be sure to read the explanations.

The answer to the first question is C. This is an important question. Is this passage about movies or fiction? Notice question stem 2. Stem 2 tells us that, in order to make a point, the author compares movies with fiction. This indicates that the author is using either movies or fiction to make a point about the other. In other words, the author is trying to tell us something about movies <u>or</u> fiction, but not both. One is more important to the author than the other. Question stems 1, 5, 6, and 7 are about fiction. Question stems 2, 3, and 4 address both movies and fiction. It seems that his point is about fiction.

The answer to the second question is A. Three of the stems deal directly with both movies and fiction. Notice the phrase 'current generation' in stem 1, indicating that *something* has recently changed in fiction. Stem 2 says that the passage compares movies with fiction. Perhaps the recent change in fiction is due to the recent phenomenon of movies. In stem 3, someone is telling beginning writers to write "as if you were a movie camera". The inference is that this will make your writing more popular. This inference is reinforced by stem 7. Stem 3 confirms that the change in fiction has something to do with movies. Stem 4 tells us that it is ironic for a movie to cause the author to read a book. 'Ironic' means that we would not expect this to happen. Thus, the author probably thinks movies have reduced peoples' interest in reading fiction. (The irony is found in the fact the this particular movie induced the author to read the fiction.)

Notice how much information can be acquired from just question stems. In order recognize this information, we had to pay close attention to exact wording.

Now write an answer to each of the seven question stems in the space below.

(**Warning:** If you read on without writing the answers, you will miss an important opportunity to improve your verbal skills. Once you read on, the effect of the exercise will be ruined.)

1.

2.

3.

4.

5.

6.

7.

Compare your answers with the actual answer choices given below, and choose a correct answer.

1.
- **A.** lacks the significance of fiction written by previous generations.
- **B.** is, as a whole, no better and no worse than fiction written by previous generations.
- **C.** brilliantly meets the particular needs of contemporary readers.
- **D.** is written by authors who show great confidence in their roles as writers.

2.
- **A.** contemporary authors have strengthened their fiction by the application of cinematic techniques.
- **B.** the film of *Under the Volcano* is bound to be more popular than the novel.
- **C.** great fiction provides a richness of language and feeling that is difficult to re-create in film.
- **D.** contemporary authors would be well advised to become screenwriters.

3.
- **I.** Gardner's approach to writing has been influenced by the competing medium of film.
- **II.** Gardner must have written screenplays at one point in his life.
- **III.** Gardner dislikes the medium of film.

- **A.** I only
- **B.** II only
- **C.** I and II only
- **D.** II and III only

4.
- **I.** seems to go against the overall point of the passage concerning fiction and film.
- **II.** implies that the film version was a box-office failure.
- **III.** hints that the author was dissatisfied with the novel.

- **A.** I only
- **B.** II only
- **C.** III only
- **D.** II and III only

5.
- **A.** prefers the quick fix of the movies.
- **B.** would be bored by a single shot of a room in a film.
- **C.** has no tolerance for movies.
- **D.** displays the attitude demanded by good fiction.

6.
- **I.** confuse and anger lovers of great literature.
- **II.** exist in stark contrast to the typical contemporary novel.
- **III.** win back some of the readers contemporary writers have lost.

- **A.** I only
- **B.** II only
- **C.** I and II only
- **D.** II and III only

7.
- **I.** competition presented by movies.
- **II.** writers themselves.
- **III.** ignorance of the public.

- **A.** I only
- **B.** II only
- **C.** I and II only
- **D.** I, II and III

Answers to these questions can be found on page 74 under "Homework". **Do not look at the answers until you are done with the lecture.**

Answer Choices

Each MCAT question has four possible answer choices. One of these will be the correct answer and the other three we will call *distracters*. Typically, when a verbal question is written, the correct answer choice is written first and then distracters are created. Because the correct answer is written to answer a specific question and a distracter is written to confuse, the two can often be distinguished without even referencing the question. In other words, with practice, a good test-taker can sometimes distinguish the correct answer among the distracters without even reading the question or the passage. This is a difficult skill to acquire and is gained only through sufficient practice.

Begin by learning to recognize typical distracter types. Among other things, effective distracters may be: a statement that displays a subtle misunderstanding of the main idea; a statement that uses the same or similar words as in the passage but is taken out of context; a true statement that does not answer the question; a statement that answers more than the question asks; a statement that relies upon information commonly considered true but not given in the passage.

In order to help you recognize distracters, we have artificially created six categories of **suspected distracters**. It is unlikely, but not impossible that the correct answer choice might also fall into one of these categories. Thus, you must use this tool as a guide to assist you in finding the correct answer, and not as an absolute test.

1) **Round-about:** a distracter that moves around the question but does not directly answer it
2) **Beyond:** a distracter whose validity relies upon information not supplied by (or information *beyond*) the passage
3) **Contrary:** a distracter that is contrary to the main idea
4) **Simpleton:** a choice that is very simple and/or easily verifiable from the passage
5) **Unintelligible:** a choice that you don't understand

Round-abouts

Round-about distracters simply don't answer the question as asked. They may be true statements. They may even concur with the passage, but they just don't offer a direct answer to the question. A Round-about is the answer you expect from a politician on a Sunday morning talk show; a lot of words were used but nothing was really said.

Beyonds

Often times, a distracter will supply information beyond the question and passage without substantiating its veracity. These distracters are called *beyonds*. When you read a beyond, you typically find yourself wondering something like "This answer sounds good, but this passage was on the economics of the post soviet union, I don't remember anything about the Russian revolution."

Beyonds can also play upon current events. A passage on AIDS may have a question with an answer choice about cloning. Cloning may be a hot topic in reality, but if it wasn't mentioned in the passage or in the question, you should be very suspicious of it being in an answer choice.

Don't confuse a *beyond* with an answer choice that directly asks you to assume information as true.

Contraries

A *contrary* distracter contradicts the main idea. If the question is not an except not or least, the answer choice is extremely unlikely to contradict the main idea. Most answer choices support the main idea in one form or another.

Simpletons

If the correct answers on the RCS were simple, direct, and straight forward, then everyone would do well. Instead, the correct answers are vague, ambiguous, and sometimes debatable. This means that an answer choice is highly suspect if it would be easily verifiable from a reading of the passage. These answer choices are called *simpletons*. Simpletons are not always the wrong answer choice, but you should be highly suspicious when you see one.

Typical of simpletons is extreme wording like *always* and *never*.

Here's a manufactured example of a simpleton:

13. In mid-afternoon in December in Montana, the author believes that the color of the sky most closely resembles:

    B. cotton balls floating on a blue sea.

If this were the answer, everyone would choose it. This is unlikely to be the correct answer.

Unintelligibles

Unintelligibles are answer choices that you don't understand. Whether it's a vocabulary word, or a concept, avoid answer choices that you don't understand. These are likely to be traps. Strangely enough, many test takers are likely to choose an answer that confuses them. This is apparently because the MCAT is a difficult test. Test writers sometimes purposely use distracters with obscure vocabulary or incomprehensible diction in order to appeal to the test taker who finds comfort in being confused. As a general rule, don't choose an answer that you don't understand unless you can positively eliminate all other choices.

Identifying the Correct Answer

Besides identifying distracters, you should become familiar with the look and feel of a typical correct answer choice.

Think about the people that write the questions for the MCAT Verbal Section. They are not the authors of the passage. They are academics. The idea is that these academics cannot hide their influence when they analyze passages and write MCAT questions. If we can learn to understand how these people think, we can more easily identify their answer choices. To do this, we must create a stereotype of the test writers. They are non-science oriented individuals who see science as a simplification of the true universe. They wallow in ambiguities, and thrive on exposing gray areas that seem to defy strict logical explanation. They love paradox and problems with no solutions. They are liberal in their political views, without being extreme. Whether or not this is true is unimportant. It works.

Typical correct answer choices contain *softeners*. Softeners are words that make the answer true under more circumstances, such as *most likely*, *seemed*, *had a tendency to*, etc. An answer choice with a softener is not necessarily correct; it is just more likely to be correct.

Summary

You have four tools for finding the correct answer (going back, main idea, question stems, and answer choices). In order to get your best MCAT score, you should use all of them. Your fourth tool is the most difficult to master. When using evaluating the answer choices for distracters, keep in mind that there are no absolutes, just suspects.

Now go back to the set of questions from the passage above, and try to answer the questions.

Stop! (Do not look at the following questions until class. If you will not be attending class, give yourself 30 minutes to complete the following set of questions.)

The following questions come from three passages. Each page represents a different passage. The passages have been removed to force you to pay attention to the questions and the answer choices. Try to answer the questions, and compare your scaled score to your normal practice MCAT score.

Passage 1

1. According to the passage, an image is a versatile tool that:

   A. is always visual, never abstract.
   B. can be either abstract or visual.
   C. is always abstract, never visual.
   D. is neither visual nor abstract.

2. An experiment found that dogs can remember a new signal for only five minutes, whereas six-year-old children can remember the same signal much longer. Based on the information in the passage, this finding is probably explained by the fact that:

   A. a human being possesses a larger store of symbolic images than a dog possesses.
   B. the human brain evolved more quickly than the brain of a dog.
   C. the children were probably much older than the dogs.
   D. most dogs are color-blind.

3. In order to defend poets from the charge that they were liars, Sidney noted that "a maker must imagine things that are not" (line 38). Sidney's point is that:

   A. a true poet must possess a powerful imagination.
   B. in order to create something, one must first imagine.
   C. poets are the most creative people in our society.
   D. imagination is not a gift unique to poets, but is possessed by all creative people.

4. In the context of the passage, the statement "if thereby we die a thousand deaths, that is the price we pay for living a thousand lives" (lines 52—54) is most likely meant to suggest that:

   A. we must guard against using our imaginations toward destructive ends.
   B. although imagination sometimes causes pain, its positive aspects outweigh its negative ones.
   C. it is possible to be too imaginative for one's own good.
   D. without imagination, the uniquely human awareness of death would not exist.

5. Which of the following findings would most *weaken* the claim that the use of symbolic imagery is unique to humans?

   A. Chimpanzees are capable of learning at least some sign language.
   B. Certain species of birds are able to migrate great distances by instinct alone.
   C. Human beings have larger frontal lobes than do other animals.
   D. Some animals have brains that are larger than human brains.

6. It has been said that language does not merely describe reality but actually helps to bring reality into existence. Which of the points made in the passage would best support this claim?

   A. To imagine means to make images and move them about in one's head.
   B. The tool that puts the human mind ahead of the animal's is imagery.
   C. There is no specific center for language in the brain of any animal except the human being.
   D. Images play out events that are not present, thereby guarding the past and creating the future.

7. According to the author, the most important images are:

   A. words.
   B. poetic images.
   C. images of the past.
   D. images of the future.

Passage 2

8. Why is the San Luis Valley site being investigated urgently?

    A. Artifacts are few in number.
    B. Artifacts are being eroded by the wind.
    C. Bison bones are few in number.
    D. Excessive rainfall is damaging the site.

9. According to the passage, which of the following activities was common to each band of Folsom Indians?

    A. Cultivating a number of different crops
    B. Eating a wide variety of wild game
    C. Interacting with other bands
    D. Making tools out of nearby rocks

10. The passage suggests that the presence of human remains, tools, and animal bones at a single location means that:

    A. bison and other animals migrated from one place to another.
    B. communal tasks were performed at the site.
    C. erosion has not yet occurred at the site.
    D. extensive interactions occurred among bands of Paleoindians.

11. Assume that a new Folsom hunter site has just been discovered in northern Texas. On the basis of the information contained in the passage, this site would most likely contain all of the following EXCEPT:

    A. clusters of bones and tools.
    B. human bones.
    C. remains of hearths.
    D. tools made of Colorado flint.

12. If a Folsom hunter site containing tools made of petrified wood were discovered in Iowa, where there is little petrified wood, this discovery would weaken which of the following conclusions made in the passage?

    I. Paleoindians hunted bison.
    II. Folsom hunters did not travel great distances.
    III. There was little trading among bands of Folsom hunters.

    A. I only
    B. III only
    C. I and II only
    D. II and III only

13. According to the passage, bands of Paleoindians did not trade between one another. What is the evidence for this statement?

    A. Tools of a band came only from local sources.
    B. Tool shapes were unique to each band.
    C. Food sources were unique to each band.
    D. Each band had its unique language and customs.

14. Given the information contained in the passage, if a large number of deer bones were discovered at the San Luis Valley site, the most likely explanation for their presence would be that the deer:

    A. accidentally died at the scene.
    B. competed with bison for food.
    C. migrated from another region.
    D. served as food for the Indians.

15. Which of the following discoveries would most strengthen the hypothesis that Folsom hunters killed the bison they ate?

    A. Bone breaks consistent with the shapes of the Folsom hunters' pointed tools
    B. No evidence of an alternative animal food source
    C. Bison bones at a Folsom site
    D. Similar accumulation of bison bones at many Folsom sites

16. If the Paleoindians had eaten small game such as rabbits instead of large game, the finding of small animal skeletons and individual tools with many edges at the same sites would LEAST support the conclusion that:

    A. certain tools had many uses.
    B. small animals made up the people's main diet.
    C. the animals were killed at the site.
    D. tools were used to prepare the animals for use.

Passage 3

17. The example concerning Galileo (lines 23—31) best supports the author's claim that:

    A. science and society usually coexist harmoniously.
    B. science works in an unpredictable manner.
    C. cultural bias limits scientific theorizing.
    D. scientific fact occasionally forces a change in cultural assumptions.

18. Based on the passage, a scientific claim has the best chance of being free from cultural influence when the claim has:

    A. much supporting evidence and much social impact.
    B. little supporting evidence and little social impact.
    C. much supporting evidence and little social impact.
    D. little supporting evidence and much social impact.

19. The author mentions the abandonment of eugenics in America and Hitler's use of arguments for sterilization and racial purification primarily to support the claim that:

    A. science is often misused.
    B. science is impartial.
    C. scientific attitudes are sometimes affected by social movements.
    D. science should avoid involvement in social issues.

20. The author believes that the view that science is an "inexorable march toward truth" (lines 66—67) is:

    A. one of the myths of science.
    B. supported by good evidence.
    C. clearly proven by the case of Galileo.
    D. accepted by most historians of science.

21. According to the author, most historians of science do NOT believe that:

    A. scientific facts lead to effective theories.
    B. most theories are developed by straightforward induction from facts.
    C. objectivity is a worthwhile goal in scientific investigation.
    D. facts are influenced by cultural assumptions.

22. When the author states that "science cannot escape its curious dialectic" (line *54)*, he is emphasizing science's:

    A. dilemma between truth and mere theories.
    B. interrelationship with social factors.
    C. quest for truth.
    D. imprecise methodology.

23. According to the author, one reason that scientists have a difficult time escaping cultural assumptions is that scientists often:

    A. formulate hypotheses that can only result in the verification of accepted beliefs.
    B. project their research findings onto society.
    C. attribute too much significance to scientific data as opposed to social belief.
    D. base theories on too much data.

Don't look at the answers yet.

Questions 1: If we look at this question and use common sense, we know that an image can be both abstract and visual. The word "versatile" in the question also helps us find the answer.

Question 2: Ask yourself "Why might a child remember a signal longer than a dog?" B, C, and D don't seem like reasonable answers. For answer B, what does it mean for a human's brain to evolve more quickly? This answer doesn't even seem to make any sense. For answer C, common sense should tell you that a six-year-old child can remember a signal longer than a dog regardless of the age of the dog. For answer choice D, the question doesn't say anything about vision. Where does color-blind come in. This is a *beyond*.

Question 3: Notice that the question asks what is meant by the quote. For this type of question, just match the answer to the quote. Answer B is a paraphrase of the quote. Sidney himself is irrelevant.

Question 4: This is the same type of question as the last. Match the answer to the quote. Notice answer choice D. This is for those who want to see things in black and white, and take the quote very literally. It also does not match the quote.

Question 5: What would weaken the claim that the use of symbolic imagery is unique to humans? An example of a non-human using symbolic imagery. A is correct.

Question 6: Here we are asked to interpret a paraphrase. Just match the paraphrase to the answer choice. "bringing reality into existence" is the same as "creating the future".

Question 7: This is difficult to answer without the passage. However, look at the other questions. Ask yourself, "What is the main idea of this passage?" It is certainly about images, symbols, and language. Which answer fits most closely? Notice that the word *image* is in all the answers except the correct one. This makes choices B, C, and D *simpletons*. A is correct.

Question 8: The word "urgently" helps to narrow down the choices to B and D. It is difficult to choose between these two without reading the passage.

Question 9: The question appears to be impossible to answer without reading the passage; however, we will find that it is easy to answer after we answer the other questions. We'll come back to it.

Question 10: This is also a difficult question to answer before we answer the others. We'll come back to it.

Question 11: The word "Texas" should stand out here. What is special about Texas? There must be something special about location and Folsom hunter sites. Looking at the answer choices, "Colorado" also stands out. What is special about Colorado? D seems like a pretty good answer. There is certainly no reason to choose any other answer. But then again, there doesn't seem to be any reason not to either. We'll come back to this one too.

Question 12: Here it is again; location! This question gives us another clue. Apparently the author believes that tools are made from material found near a site because if tools were found that were not made from material near the site, this would somehow weaken the author's argument. Here, it makes sense that if the author argued for either II or III, both would be weakened. There doesn't seem to be any reason why choice I would be weakened. B or D must be the answer. But wait, if the author thought that Folsom hunters did travel great distances, then they might have carried tools with them, and III would not be weakened. Therefore, D must be the answer.

Question 9 revisited: Now we know that the answer to question 9 must be D.

Question 10 revisited: Now we know that D must be wrong. Notice the word "single" emphasizing the importance that the tools appear together. Choice B also addresses this togetherness with the word "communal". A and C don't seem to have a mechanism which would explain them. The correct answer is B.

Question 11 revisited: Clearly, if tools must be made from nearby materials, "tools made from Colorado flint" would not be found at a site in "northern Texas". D is correct.

Question 13: This question even tells you part of the answer to question 12. Answer A just confirms what we've already discovered. A is correct.

Question 14: This question can be answered using the other questions as background. The passage is about the Folsom hunters. Only D incorporates this into its answer. The main idea is always the best choice.

Question 15: The question asks for something that would prove (show) that the hunters killed the bison that they ate. In other words, the question wants something that would show that they didn't scavenge the bison after finding them dead, but they actually killed them. Choice A shows that the bison were killed with tools made by the hunters. Choice A is also the only choice that seems consistent with a main idea that apparently has to do with tools.

Question 16: Notice that the question emphasizes small versus large. The only answer choice that addresses this emphasis is choice C. If the game were small, the hunters could have carried their prey to the site.

Question 17: If you know that Galileo was forced by the church to recant his theories, you know that A is wrong. This information also seems to suggest C or D. We'll come back to this one.

Question 18: This is just common sense. Now we know what the passage is about.

Question 19: Certainly B is wrong. The problem with both A and D is that the example includes a 'good thing' about science, the abandonment of eugenics, and a bad thing about science, Hitler use of it. (Eugenics is the creation of a the perfect race through breeding.) A and D suggest that both are bad, so they are the wrong answer choices. C is correct.

Question 20: This is a perfect example of a non-MCAT verbal thought: "science is an inexorable march toward truth." Verbal is ambiguous, not absolute. This is extremely unlikely to be the belief of an author in the Verbal Section. A is clearly the correct answer because it is so MCAT-like.

Question 21: The main idea is about the relationship between social events and science. Clearly B is correct. B is also very MCAT-like in its non-absolutism.

Question 22: B is main idea; it must be correct. A and D are beyonds. C is not MCAT-like.

Question 23: C and D don't make sense; they seem to contradict the logic of the question. A answers the question better than B because B has science affecting society as opposed to the way the question has society affecting science.

Question 17 revisited: We were stuck between C and D. Unfortunately, we're still stuck. We'll have to just guess, or read the passage. We still get at least an MCAT score of 12.

The answers to these stand alone questions can be found on page 74 under "Stand Alones".

This exercise is not to convince you not to read the passage. You should always read the passage. It should show you that there is a large amount of information in the questions and answer choices. If you scored higher without reading the passage, then you probably haven't been taking advantage of the wealth of information in the questions and answer choices.

Lecture 3:
The Main Idea

The main idea is a summary of the passage in one or two sentences. It should reflect the author's opinion (if presented or implied), and it should emphasize minor topics to the same extent as they are emphasized in the passage. It is not a list of topics discussed in the passage nor an outline of those topics. It is a statement about the passage topics, and includes the author's opinion.

In one form or another, 90% of the Verbal Section questions will concern the main idea. Notice that the main idea cannot be found by going back to the passage and searching for details. You must concentrate on the main idea while you read the entire passage. If you read for detail, if you try to remember what you have read rather than process what you are reading, you will have to guess at 90% of the questions.

It is important to have a clear concept of the main idea before reading any questions. MCAT Verbal section questions are designed to take your inchoate thoughts concerning the passage and subtly redirect them away from the true main idea. Each successive question embellishes on insidious pseudo-themes steering unwary followers into an abyss from which there is no return. Like a faithful paladin, your clearly stated main idea unmasks these impostors and leads you toward the holy grail of Verbal Section perfection.

Writing the main idea on paper is an important step toward improving your ability to find the main idea; however, it requires too much time while taking the exam. Instead, the day after taking a practice exam, go back to each passage and write out the main idea. While taking the exam, make a 20 second pause after reading a passage, and construct the main idea in your head.

Most students resist writing down their main idea until they are halfway through the course and the materials. At this point they begin to realize how important the main idea is. Unfortunately, they must start from scratch and begin writing down the main idea with only four weeks until the MCAT. Don't do this. Start now by writing down the main idea. It's very painful at first, but it will get easier, and it will dramatically improve your score.

Constructing the Main Idea

A good main idea can be formed as follows: 1) After reading the passage, write down the main topics. Each topic should be from one to four words. 2) From these topics, choose the most important two or three, and write a short phrase relating them to each other and the passage. 3) Now lengthen the phrase into one or two sentences which still concern the most important topics but incorporate the other topics as well. Be sure to include the author's opinion if it was given or implied. Try to emphasize each topic to the same extent to which it was emphasized in the passage. This is your main idea.

Confidence

Often on the MCAT, passages seem incomprehensible. Don't get bent! Remember, most questions are answered correctly by more than 60% of test-takers, and only two or three are answered incorrectly by less than 40%, so no group of questions will be that difficult. Have the confidence to keep reading. **<u>Don't reread a line or paragraph over and over until you master it.</u>** If a line or paragraph is incomprehensible to you, then it is probably incomprehensible to everyone else, and understanding it will not help your score. Instead, continue reading until you get to something that you do understand. Just get the general sense of what the author is trying to say. Chances are good that this will be enough to answer all the questions. Remember, the passage is only one tool out of four to help you answer the questions.

Know Your Author

You must become familiar with the author. Who is he or she? Is the author young or old; rich or poor; male or female; conservative or liberal? Do you love or hate this author? Take a guess. Create a picture of the author in your mind. Use your prejudices to stereotype the author. Your harsh judgment of the author is everything to understanding what he is trying to say. The better you understand the author, the easier will be the questions. Read with emotion and judge harshly.

Now that you know the author intimately, when you get to a question, ask yourself "If this author were right here in front of me, how would he answer this question?" The way that the author would answer the question, is always, without exception, the correct answer.

Ignore the details and See the Big Picture

There is no reason to remember the details of a passage. They can be found in seconds, and are rarely important to answering a question. Instead, focus on the big picture. Ask yourself "What is the author trying to say to me? What's his beef?" The author's 'beef' will be the main idea, and the key to answering 90% of the questions.

**The section that follows includes material from the MCAT Practice Test 1/Practice Items. These materials are reprinted with permission of the Association of American Medical Colleges (AAMC).

Stop Here Until Class! (Do not look at the following passage and questions until class. If you will not be attending class, read the passage in two minutes and 30 seconds, and answer the questions which follow.)

Passage

It is roughly a century since European art began to experience its first significant defections from the standards of painting and sculpture that we inherit from the early Renaissance. Looking back now across a long succession of innovative movements and stylistic revolutions, most of us have little trouble recognizing that such aesthetic orthodoxies of the past as the representative convention, exact anatomy and optical perspective, the casement-window canvas, along with the repertory of materials and subject matters we associate with the Old Masters—that all this makes up not "art" itself in any absolute sense, but something like a *school* of art, one great tradition among many. We acknowledge the excellence which a Raphael or Rembrandt could achieve within the canons of that school; but we have grown accustomed to the idea that there are other aesthetic visions of equal validity. Indeed, innovation in the arts has become a convention in its own right with us, a "tradition of the new," to such a degree that there are critics to whom it seems to be intolerable that any two painters should paint alike. We demand radical originality, and often confuse it with quality.

Yet what a jolt it was to our great-grandparents to see the certainties of the academic tradition melt away before their eyes. How distressing, especially for the academicians, who were the guardians of a classic heritage embodying time-honored techniques and standards whose perfection had been the labor of genius. Suddenly they found art as they understood it being rejected by upstarts who were unwilling to let a single premise of the inherited wisdom stand unchallenged, or so it seemed. Now, with a little hindsight, it is not difficult to discern continuities where our predecessors saw only ruthless disjunctions. To see, as well, that the artistic revolutionaries of the past were, at their best, only opening our minds to a more global conception of art which demanded a deeper experience of light, color, and form. Through their work, too, the art of our time has done much to salvage the values of the primitive and childlike, the dream, the immediate emotional response, the life of fantasy, and the transcendent symbol.

In our own day, much the same sort of turning point has been reached in the history of science. It is as if the aesthetic ground pioneered by the artists now unfolds before us as a new ontological awareness. We are at a moment when the reality to which scientists address themselves comes more and more to be recognized as but one segment of a far broader spectrum. Science, for so long regarded as our single valid picture of the world, now emerges as, also, a school: a *school of consciousness*, beside which alternative realities take their place.

There are, so far, only fragile and scattered beginnings of this perception. They are still the subterranean history of our time. How far they will carry toward liberating us from the orthodox world view of the technocratic establishment is still doubtful. These days, many gestures of rebellion are subtly denatured, adjusted, and converted into oaths of allegiance. In our society at large, little beyond submerged unease challenges the lingering authority of science and technique, that dull ache at the bottom of the soul we refer to when we speak (usually too glibly) of an "age of anxiety," an "age of longing."

Answer the following questions without going back to the passage. If you don't know the answer, guess.

YOU MAY NOT LOOK AT THE PASSAGE!

Is the author male or female?
Does the author have long or short hair?
How old is the author?
What political party is the author a member of?
Would the author prefer a wild party or a night at the opera?
Do you think you would like the author?
What does the author do for a living?

These are the types of questions that you should be able to answer with prejudice if you have read the passage the way you should. If you can answer these questions, you have compared the author to people of your past and categorized the author accordingly. This means that you have a better understanding of who the author is, and how he would answer the MCAT questions about his own passage.

The previous questions were asked to make you realize how you should be trying to understand the author. You should not be asking yourself these questions on a real MCAT. Here are some questions that you should ask yourself on a real MCAT:

YOU MAY NOT LOOK AT THE PASSAGE!

If the author were sitting in front of you, would he or she want to discuss science or art?
What emotion, if any, is the author feeling?
Is the author a scientist?
Is the author conservative, liberal, or somewhere in the middle?

The answers to these questions are unequivocal. This author is discussing science, not art. Art is used as a lengthy, nearly incomprehensible introduction to make a point about science. The author doesn't even begin discussing the main idea until the beginning of the third paragraph. "In our own day, much the same sort of turning point has been reached in the history of science." When you read this, you should have been startled. You should have been thinking "Where did science come from? I thought we were talking about some esoteric art history crap that I really wasn't understanding." This one sentence should have said to you "Ahaa! That other stuff was appetizer, now the author is going to discuss his real interest." Notice that it is at the beginning of the third paragraph that the writing actually becomes intelligible. In other words, the second two paragraphs are much easier to read. This is because the author is interested in this topic and knows what he wants to say. The art stuff was a poorly written introduction and the author had not thought it through with any clarity. If you spent lots of time rereading the first two paragraphs, trying to master them, you wasted your time. The author didn't even master them; how could you?

The author is frustrated and possibly even bitter. He is so angry, that he is name-calling. For instance, he calls the scientific community "the technocratic establishment". The tone of the passage is like that of a whining child. He blames scientists for being too conservative and thus creating "an age of anxiety", as if the anxiety of most people would be relieved if scientists were less practical. In the last sentence, he even blames us, his reader, for not taking *his* issue more seriously. The author is positively paranoid. Notice that his adversaries move against him "subtly" as if trying to hide their evil intentions. They take "oaths of allegiance" like some NAZI cult. This is way over done when you consider that the guy's only complaint is that science isn't liberal enough in its approach.

The author is certainly not a scientist. First of all, he writes like a poet not a scientist: "orthodox world view of the technocratic establishment", "subterranean history of our time", "gestures of rebellion subtly denatured". Secondly, his whole point is that he is upset with scientists. (An entire separate argument can be made that his point results from his misunderstanding of how science progresses.) And finally, he talks like a member of some pyramid cult, not a scientist: "alternative realities" and "ontological awareness". This author probably flunked high school physics and just can't get over it.

The author is certainly liberal, or antiestablishment. He talks about "liberating us" and "rebellion" among other things.

Now, with this understanding of the author, answer the questions on the next page.

YOU MAY NOT LOOK AT THE PASSAGE!

1. The author believes that in "the subterranean history of our time" (line 53-55) we find the beginnings of a:

    A. renewal of allegiance to traditional values.
    B. redefinition of art.
    C. redefinition of science.
    D. single valid picture of the world.

2. The author compares art and science mainly in support of idea that:

    A. The conventions of science, like those of art, are now beginning to be recognized as but one segment of a far broader spectrum.
    B. aesthetic orthodoxies of the past, unlike scientific orthodoxies of the present, make up only one tradition among many.
    C. artistic as well as scientific revolutionaries open our minds to a more global conception of art.
    D. artists of the past have provided inspiration to the scientists of the present.

3. The two kinds of art discussed in the passage are the:

    A. aesthetic and the innovative.
    B. dull and the shocking.
    C. traditional and the innovative.
    D. representative and the traditional.

4. The author's statement "How far [new perceptions of science] will carry toward liberating us from the orthodox world view of the technocratic establishment is still doubtful" (lines 54-56) assumes that the:

    A. technocratic establishment is opposed to scientific inquiry.
    B. traditional perception of science is identical to the world view of the technocratic establishment.
    C. current perceptions of science are identical to those of art.
    D. technocratic establishment has the same world view as the artistic revolutionaries of the past.

5. Which of the following concepts does the author illustrate with specific examples?

    A. Scientific innovations of the present
    B. Scientific innovations of the past
    C. Aesthetic innovations of the present
    D. Aesthetic orthodoxies of the past

6. The claim that the unease mentioned in line 59 is "submerged" most directly illustrates the idea that:

    A. our great-grandparents were jolted by the collapse of academic certainty.
    B. we have grown accustomed to the notion that there is more than one valid aesthetic vision.
    C. so far, new perceptions of science are only fragile and scattered.
    D. the authority of science is rapidly being eroded.

7. Based on the information in the passage, the author would most likely claim that someone who did NOT agree with his view of science was:

    A. dishonest.
    B. conformist.
    C. rebellious.
    D. imaginative.

8. Based on information in the passage, which of the following opinions could most reasonably be ascribed to the author?

    A. It is misguided to rebel against scientific authority.
    B. The world views of other disciplines may have something valuable to teach the scientific community.
    C. Art that rebels against established traditions cannot be taken seriously.
    D. The main cause of modern anxiety and longing is our rash embrace of new scientific and artistic theories.

9. Adopting the author's views as presented in the passage would most likely mean acknowledging that:

    A. it is not a good idea to accept traditional beliefs simply because they are traditional.
    B. we must return to established artistic and scientific values.
    C. the future is bleak for today's artists and scientists.
    D. the scientific community has given us little of benefit.

48

Don't worry about the correct answers yet.

YOU MAY NOT LOOK AT THE PASSAGE YET!

The first thing to notice is that only question 5 requires any information from the first two paragraphs, and question 5 was a question about detail, not concept. This is because the first two paragraphs are not about the main idea.

The second thing to notice is that none of the questions require us to go back to the passage, even though some refer us to specific line numbers. All but question 5 are answerable directly from the main idea. Question 5 is a detailed question, but before you run back to the passage to find the answer, look at the possibilities. The chances are that you remembered Raphael and Rembrandt from the first paragraph. These are specific examples of "aesthetic orthodoxies of the past".

Notice that many of the questions can be rephrased to say "The author thinks _____." This is typical of an MCAT passage, and that's why you must "know your author".

Questions 1: Forget about the quote for a moment. Simplify the question to say "The author thinks that we find the beginnings of a:" Answer C is the main idea. Certainly the author would disagree with A, B, and D.

Questions 2: "The author thinks:" that science is like art, and that conventions of both are but part of a larger spectrum. B says science is not like art; the opposite of what the author thinks. C says that scientific revolutionaries are changing science; the author is frustrated because this is not really happening. D says scientists of the present are opening their minds to new ideas; the author complains that they are not.

Question 3: The main idea of the passage contains the theme of traditional vs. innovative.

Questions 4: Ignore the quotes until you need them. Without the quotes, the questions says "The author's statement assumes that the:" In other words, "The author thinks _____." C and D are exactly opposite to what the author thinks. Answer A plays a common game on the MCAT. They take the authors view to far. They want you to think "the author doesn't like the scientists; therefore, he thinks the scientists can't even do science." Even this author wouldn't go that far. A is incorrect. Answer B requires you to realize that the "technocratic establishment" is conservative.

Question 6: Answer D is out because it disagrees with the main idea, and C is the only answer that supports the main idea. However, this question is best answered by comparing the answer choices with the question. The question asks for an example of "submerged unease". "jolted" in answer choice A certainly doesn't describe submerged unease. "grown accustomed" in answer choice B certainly does not describe submerged unease. Answer choice C could describe submerged unease, and it does describe the main idea. It is the best answer.

Question 7: The author is rebellious and imaginative. If you disagree with him, he thinks you are a conformist, which, by the way, is worse than dishonest as far as he's concerned.

Question 8: "The author thinks _____." The whole point of the intro is to say that the scientific community should learn from the discipline of art.

Question 9: "The author thinks _____." The author is a rebel. He thinks you should always question authority. Notice choice D is another example of taking things too far. No sane individual could argue that science has provided little benefit. Answer choice C would be incorrect even if it had not included 'artists'. It would have been too extreme.

NOW YOU MAY LOOK AT THE PASSAGE.

Hopefully, we have demonstrated the power of knowing the author and understanding the main idea. Remember to use all four of your tools, and, most importantly, read and answer questions with confidence.

If you have problems, go back to the basics of this manual. Figure out what part of our strategy and tactics you aren't using, and use it.

Good luck!

STOP!

Do not look at these exams until class.

30-minute
In-class Exam
for Lecture 1

In July 1589, the governing council of Amsterdam…
…announced itself interested in establishing a "house where all vagabonds, evildoers, rascals and the like could be imprisoned"…

5 …the Amsterdam Tugthuis, which opened its doors on the Heiligeweg in 1595 [became a stop] on any tourist itinerary of Amsterdam. Ushered there by burgomasters and magistrates, a procession of visitors from England, France, Italy, Germany, Scandinavia and
10 even Hungary all recorded their visits there… Many of them were struck by the formidable system of disciplinary punishments that backed up the house regime… On November 13, 1618, no fewer than twenty prisoners (or about a quarter of the inmates) were
15 whipped in one day for their obstinacy. Worse was the contraption that bent the prisoner across a bench, with his head in a vise, while the birch was applied to the body. As grim as these "correctives" were, a good number of travelers mentioned another punishment for
20 the incorrigibly idle so sinister as to defy credulity. This was the drowning cell or "water house." Jean de Parival's terse reference in 1662 is typical of the laconic—but emphatic—description of this dramatic frightener: "If they do not want to work they are
25 tethered like asses and are put in a cellar that is filled with water so that they must partly empty it by pumping if they do not wish to drown."

It is difficult not to blink in disbelief in reading this. But caravans of tourists from the early to the late
30 seventeenth century all pointed it out in their accounts…even Joseph Marshall, the economics writer…congratulated the magistrates on so "admirable a contrivance."

For all his sharp-eyed empiricism on so many other
35 aspects of Holland, Marshall's report of the drowning cell is suspiciously inaccurate. He was led to suppose that "by law" the incorrigibly idle were supposed to drown if they did not use the pump to the best of their ability. Yet at about the same date…the official
40 historian of Amsterdam, Johan Wagenaar, who gave a thorough account of the punishment of offenders, dismissed the cell as pure hearsay…Travelers' accounts, many (though not all) secondhand, should be offset by the eloquent silence of contemporary Dutch
45 sources, including city descriptions like the *Beschryving der Stat Amsterdam* of 1665 by Tobias van Domselaer and Olfert Dapper…

Was the drowning cell a bizarre fable, a sadistic fantasy, concocted from half-digested gobbets of
50 hearsay?…For all [the] gaps in our knowledge, the possibility of this cold-blooded experiment in behaviorist persuasion having functioned at some time

cannot be entirely dismissed. There is at least one seventeenth-century Dutch source…that gave a detailed
55 account of the cell…

When taken together with the interest shown by the magistrates of Danzig in…this device, and their attempt to engineer a modified version of it (with rope and well), there seems more than a shred of possibility that
60 the drowning cell did, for a while at least, carry out its work of salutary intimidation. But supposing it was only a popular and perennially repeated myth, would that obviate its historical importance? Not, at any rate, in the realm of culture, where belief and utterance were
65 as potent social realities as tangible action…And at a time when all manner of gruesome public retribution was taken—slit noses, wheel-broken bodies, bored tongues, even pierced eyes—the notion of the traumatic coercion of the lazy would not have seemed particularly
70 barbaric. So if the story of the drowning cell seemed to the parade of well-to-do travelers entirely of a piece with Amsterdam's other provision for the delinquent, how much more compelling would have been even a rumor to those of the common people who might
75 expect a spell in the house on the Heiligeweg.

1. Assuming it existed, what was the purpose of the drowning cell?

   A. To execute incorrigible prisoners
   B. To test the faith of those accused of hearsay
   C. To encourage the lazy to work
   D. To frighten the enemies of Holland

2. What is the author's attitude towards the merits of a drowning cell?

   A. It is preferable to physical punishments, such as whipping, because permanent harm is not done.
   B. It is preferable to barbaric punishments, such as eye-piercing, because it is intended to reform rather than punish.
   C. It is preferable to common punishments, such as imprisonment, because its unusual nature causes it to be widely publicized, acting as a deterrent.
   D. It should not be used because of its excessive cruelty.

GO ON TO THE NEXT PAGE.

3. The accounts of Marshall and Wagenaar conflict. Based on the evidence presented in the passage, how could the conflict be reconciled?

A. Marshall probably made up the story in order to support his economic theories.
B. The Dutch government had Wagenaar under strict orders to cover up this violation of human rights.
C. Marshall believed a rumor that was actually untrue.
D. At the time of Marshall's visit, the "water house" was in use, but Wagenaar, writing one hundred years later, did not know of its existence.

4. According to the passage, what was the prevailing attitude of most sixteenth and seventeenth century tourists to the Tugthuis?

A. Shock at the substandard treatment of the prisoners
B. Fear for their own safety in such a repressive state
C. Skepticism at the lies of the Dutch
D. Admiration for an innovative form of correction

5. If the drowning chamber was a "perennially repeated myth" (line 62) encouraged by the Dutch government, what purpose might it have served?

A. It made other punishments, such as nose-slitting, seem mild by comparison.
B. It deterred petty crime, such as pickpocketting.
C. It deterred high crimes, such as treason.
D. It frightened foreign diplomats.

6. Which of the following discoveries, if true, would most strongly SUPPORT the actual existence of the drowning chamber?

A. A directive from the governing council of Amsterdam to the warden of the Tugthuis to deny all knowledge of the water house
B. Reports by foreign visitors of a similar device in Prague
C. Recovery of the "contraption" described in lines 15-16
D. Records from Tugthuis indicating that an average of twelve prisoners per year died while in the prison

7. Jean de Parival is most likely a:

A. former inmate of Tugthuis.
B. social historian.
C. priest.
D. middle-class foreigner.

8. Which of the following pieces of evidence for the actual existence of the drowning cell is mentioned in the passage?

I. Foreign accounts
II. A Dutch account
III. Physical evidence
IV. Indirect evidence based on actions taken in other countries

A. I only
B. I and II only
C. I, III, and IV only.
D. I, II, and IV only.

9. The author's attitude toward seventeenth century systems of punishment and reform can best be described as:

A. amused.
B. angered.
C. enthused.
D. appalled.

10. Which of the following would NOT be an example of "belief and utterance" as "potent social realities" (lines 64-65)?

A. a poor person wishing for a winning lottery ticket and winning the lottery on the next day
B. a political party which changed its name in order to disassociate itself from past scandals
C. a king making laws based upon his divine right
D. a stock which increased in value because of a favorable comment by an economist

Passage II (Questions 11-17)

On top of the…social layers of blue- and white-collar workers who comprise the working class and make up 85-90 percent of the population, there sits a very small social upper class which comprises at most 0.5 percent
5   of the population and has a very different lifestyle and source of income from the rest of us. Many Americans are not even aware of the existence of this upper class. They are used to thinking of the highly paid and highly visible doctors, architects, television actors, corporate
10 managers, writers, government officials and experts who stand between the working class and the upper class as the highest level of the social pecking order. The "rich people," if they come to mind at all, are thought of as a few wealthy eccentrics, such as Howard
15 Hughes, who happened to strike it rich; or as the occasional wealthy families, such as the Rockefellers or Mellons or Du Ponts, which are thought to be a remnant of another age; or as the handful of playboys or jet setters who are bent on squandering the little that
20 remains from once-significant family fortunes.

But "the rich" in the United States are not a handful of discontented eccentrics, jet setters and jaded scions who have been pushed aside by the rise of corporations and governmental bureaucracies. They are instead full-
25 fledged members of a thriving social class which is as alive and well as it has ever been. Members of this privileged class, according to sociological and journalistic studies, live in secluded neighborhoods and well-guarded apartment complexes, send their children
30 to private boarding schools, announce their teen-age daughters to the world by means of debutante teas and gala ballroom dances, play backgammon and dominoes at their exclusive social clubs and travel all over the world on their numerous junkets and vacations…

35 There is also in America, as different types of studies show, an extremely distorted distribution of wealth…For selected years between 1953 and 1969, the top one percent of the population has owned between 25 percent and 30 percent of all privately held material
40 wealth …these figures, it should be stressed, are considered conservative estimates, for good information on this touchy topic is hard to obtain…

It is not hard for most of us to imagine that the small social upper class uncovered in sociological research is
45 made up of the top wealthholders revealed in wealth and income studies…it is [also] possible to do empirical studies linking the one category to the other…The first systematic studies along this line were reported by sociologist E. Digby Blatzell, who showed
50 that the wealthiest people of Philadelphia and also the people who send their children to expensive private schools, belong to exclusive social clubs and list in the "blue book" of the upper class, the *Social Register*…

In most countries, it would be taken for granted that a
55 social upper class with a highly disproportionate amount of wealth and income is a ruling class with domination over the government…

Not so in the United States today. In a nation that has always denied the existence of social classes and
60 class conflict, and overestimated the degree of social mobility, systematic information on the persistent inequality of wealth and income tends to get lost from public and academic debate. Besides, most social scientists, being of a pluralist persuasion, believe that
65 many different groups, including organized labor, farmers, consumers and middle-class environmentalists, have a hand in political debates…there is no such thing as a ruling class in America, or so we are assured by leading academicians, journalists and other public
70 figures.

11. The author's central thesis is that:

A.   Social mobility in the U.S. is not as prevalent as most believe.
B.   Something must be done about the small group of decadent rich that virtually control the U.S. government.
C.   The United States has a wealthy ruling class that goes largely unnoticed by the rest of the population.
D.   The wealthiest of the upper class are squandering their once-significant fortunes on debutante teas and expensive junkets.

12. The tone of the passage is best described as:

A.   matter-of-fact
B.   mildly critical
C.   deeply concerned
D.   controlled anger

GO ON TO THE NEXT PAGE.

54

13. For which of the following does the author cite no evidence?

    A. Many Americans are not even aware of the existence of the ruling class.
    B. The top economic class comprises the same people as the top social class.
    C. In America, there is a very disproportionate distribution of wealth.
    D. Members of the privileged class live in secluded neighborhoods.

14. Which of the following would most strongly *challenge* the view of the author that a ruling class of extremely wealthy citizens exists in the United States?

    A. A survey demonstrating that most people are aware that a small group of U.S. citizens owns a disproportionately large share of the material wealth.
    B. The discovery that in some other country, the ruling class does not comprise the wealthiest citizens.
    C. A study that found that political candidates supported by the wealthiest citizens generally lose.
    D. A study which found that the number of millionaires in the United States is increasing.

15. Which of the following is NOT mentioned as an activity of the privileged class?
    A. playing dominoes
    B. taking vacations in foreign countries
    C. enrolling their children in private schools
    D. running for public office

16. What does the author mean by the phrase "conservative estimates" in line 41?

    A. Probably more than one percent of the population holds 25 to 30 percent of the nation's material wealth.
    B. Probably the top one percent of the population owns more than 30 percent of the nation's material wealth.
    C. Probably less than one percent of the population owns less than 25 percent of the nation's material wealth.
    D. Probably more than one percent of the population holds more than one percent of the nation's material wealth.

17. Suppose a study found that the wealthiest 1% of American citizens favored social programs such as welfare, job training, and free education to a much greater extent than members of the "professional class" described in lines 8-12. How would that affect the author's subsequent arguments?

    A. It would support the claim that the United States overestimates the degree of social mobility.
    B. It would challenge the claim that the distribution of wealth in the United States is extremely distorted.
    C. It would challenge the claim that the privileged class is thriving.
    D. It would have no direct effect on the subsequent arguments.

GO ON TO THE NEXT PAGE.

Passage III (Questions 18-23)

Mahzaria Banaji doesn't fit anybody's idea of a racist. A psychology professor at Yale University, she studies stereotypes for a living. And as a woman and a member of a minority ethnic group, she has felt
5 firsthand the sting of discrimination. Yet when she took one of her own tests of unconscious bias "I showed very strong prejudices." she said, "It was truly a disconcerting experience." And an illuminating one. When Banaji was in graduate school in the early 1980s,
10 theories about stereotypes were concerned only with their explicit expression: outright and unabashed racism, sexism, anti-Semitism. But in the years since, a new approach to stereotypes has shattered that simple notion. The bias Banaji and her colleagues are studying
15 is something far more subtle, and more insidious: what's known as automatic or implicit stereotyping, which, they find, we do all the time without knowing it. Though out-and-out bigotry may be on the decline, says Banaji, "if anything, stereotyping is a bigger problem
20 than we ever imagined."

Previously researchers who studied stereotyping had simply asked people to record their feelings about minority groups and had used their answers as an index of their attitudes. Psychologists now understand that
25 these conscious replies are only half the story. How progressive a person seems to be on the surface bears little or no relation to how prejudiced he or she is on an unconscious level—so that a bleeding-heart, liberal might harbor just as many biases as a neo-Nazi
30 skinhead.

The test that exposed Banaji's hidden biases—and that this writer took as well, with equally dismaying results—is typical of the ones used by automatic stereotype researchers. It presents the subject with a
35 series of positive or negative adjectives, each paired with a characteristically "white" or "black" name. As the name and word appear together on a computer screen, the person taking the test presses a key, indicating whether the word is good or bad.
40 Meanwhile, the computer records the speed of each response.

A glance at subjects' response times reveals a startling phenomenon: Most people who participate in the experiment—even some African-Americans—
45 respond more quickly when a positive word is paired with a white name or a negative word with a black name. Because our minds are more accustomed to making these associations, says Banaji, they process them more rapidly. Though the words and names aren't
50 subliminal, they are presented so quickly that a subject's ability to make deliberate choices is diminished—allowing his or her underlying as-sumptions to show through. The same technique can be used to measure stereotypes about many different social
55 groups, such as homosexuals, women, and the elderly.

Research done after World War II concluded that stereotypes were used only by a particular type of person: rigid, repressed, authoritarian. …The cognitive approach refused to let the rest of us off the hook. It
60 made the simple but profound point that we all use categories—of people, places, things—to make sense of the world around us. "Our ability to categorize and evaluate is an important part of human intelligence." says Banaji. "Without it, we couldn't survive." But
65 stereotypes are too much of a good thing. In the course of stereotyping, a useful category—say, women—becomes freighted with additional associations, usually negative. "Stereotypes are categories that have gone too far," says John Bargh, Ph.D., of New York
70 University. "When we use stereotypes, we take in the gender, the age, the color of the skin of the person before us, and our minds respond with messages that say hostile, stupid, slow, weak. Those qualities aren't out there in the environment. They don't reflect
75 reality."

Though a small minority of scientists argues that stereotypes are usually accurate and can be relied upon without reservations, most disagree—and vehemently. "Even if there is a kernel of truth in the stereotype,
80 you're still applying a generalization about a group to an individual, which is always incorrect," says Bargh. Accuracy aside, some believe that the use of stereotypes is simply unjust. "In a democratic society, people should be judged as individuals and not as
85 members of a group," Banaji argues. "Stereotyping flies in the face of that ideal."

---

18. Based on the passage, with which of the following statements would the author of the passage most likely agree?

   A. A bleeding heart liberal may be just as likely to commit a bias crime as a neo-Nazi skinhead.
   B. Although unpleasant, stereotypes have a necessary place in society.
   C. Human mores should be guided by modern scientific theories rather than traditional thinking.
   D. A democratic form of government is preferable to socialism.

GO ON TO THE NEXT PAGE.

19. The author's description of scientific opinion concerning the reliability of stereotypes (lines 76-78) can best be described as:

    A. fair and impartial.
    B. subtly self-serving.
    C. largely uninformed.
    D. grossly overstated.

20. Which of the following would most WEAKEN Dr. Banaji's hypothesis as derived from the test results?

    A. Some of the subjects tested had slower reflexes than others.
    B. Some subjects that admitted being racist were found by the test to hold fewer prejudices than those that claimed they were not racist.
    C. Most subjects tested were unable to distinguish between white and black names.
    D. All subjects, including those shown not to be racist, vehemently disagreed with their test results.

21. According to one social scientist, "Although negative stereotypes are widely held throughout society, and translate into lower wages for minorities, stereotypes during wartime translate into an effective fighting machine." This social scientist probably:

    A. disapproves of affirmative action laws applied to the military.
    B. believes that wartime propaganda does not effect peacetime minority hiring practices.
    C. believes that minority workers currently receive less pay for the same job.
    D. believes that positive stereotyping between nations can prevent wars.

22. If true, which of the following would most WEAKEN Banaji's conclusion that "In a democratic society, people should be judged as individuals and not as members of a group"?

    A. Efforts to unite African-American politicians as a single effective voting block have largely failed.
    B. Political organizations founded upon racist principles thrive in certain parts of the country.
    C. Most elected officials vote along party lines regardless of their personal feelings.
    D. Studies show that communist societies promote individualistic behavior more strongly than democratic societies.

23. The author of the passage specifically mentions her own stereotypical view of:

    A. black, urban youths.
    B. successful, white males.
    C. homosexuals.
    D. educated, minority women.

STOP. IF YOU FINISH BEFORE TIME IS CALLED, CHECK YOUR WORK. YOU MAY GO BACK TO ANY QUESTION IN THIS TEST BOOKLET.

STOP.

30-minute
In-class Exam
for Lecture 2

Passage I (Questions 24-30)

The Kennedy experiment can be viewed as a test of a moderate version of the psychological theory that seeks to use symbolic gestures as unilateral initiatives to reduce tension to get at other factors, leading towards
5   multilateral negotiations.

The first step was a speech by President John F. Kennedy…in which he outlined "A Strategy of Peace." While it is not known to what degree the President or his advisors were moved by a psychological theory, the
10 speech clearly met a condition of this theory—it set the *context* for the unilateral initiatives to follow. As any concrete measure can be interpreted in a variety of ways, it is necessary to spell out the general state of mind these steps attempt to communicate.

15 The President called attention to the dangers of nuclear war and took a reconciliatory tone toward the Soviet Union in his address. He said that "constructive changes" in the Soviet Union "might bring within reach solutions which now seem beyond us." He stated that
20 "our problems are man-made…and can be solved by man." Coming eight months after the 1962 Cuban crisis, when the United States and Russia stood "eyeball to eyeball," such statements marked a decisive change in American attitudes. United States policies, the
25 President added, must be so constructed "that it becomes in the Communist interest to agree to a genuine peace," which was a long way from the prevailing sentiment that there was little the United States could do, so long as the Soviet Union did not
30 change…Nor did the President imply that all the blame for the cold war rested with the other side; he called on Americans to "re-examine" their attitudes toward the cold war.

Beyond merely delivering a speech, the President
35 announced the first unilateral initiative—the United States was stopping all nuclear tests in the atmosphere and would not resume them unless another country did. This, it should be noted, was basically a psychological gesture and not a unilateral arms limitation step. The
40 United States at that time was believed to command about five times the means of delivery of the Soviet Union and to have them much better protected, and had conducted about twice as many nuclear tests, including a recent large round of testing. American experts
45 believed that it would take about one to two years before the information from these tests was finally digested, that in all likelihood little was to be gained from additional testing even after that date, and that if testing proved to be necessary it could be conducted in
50 other environments, particularly underground. Thus, in effect, the President used the termination of testing as a psychological gesture.

24. Which of the following would the author consider most similar in function to the termination of atmospheric nuclear testing discussed in this passage?

  A. A negotiated arms reduction treaty signed by the United States and the Soviet Union.

  B. A decision by the United States to unilaterally cut the emission of greenhouse gasses by 20%, despite the substantial economic hardship it would cause.

  C. An announcement by a car company that it would improve the fuel economy of its cars to meet the demand of environmentalists, using a new technology that would not increase the production cost of the cars.

  D. A promise by a terrorist that he would release all of his hostages in exchange for the release of certain prisoners held by the government.

25. According to the theory given in the passage, what did President Kennedy hope to accomplish by discontinuing atmospheric testing?

  A. He hoped to trick the Soviets into giving up something of value.

  B. He wanted to improve his political standing at home.

  C. He wanted to give his scientists time to analyze the recent tests.

  D. He hoped it would lead to substantive peace treaties.

26. Which of the following would most strongly *challenge* the "psychological" explanation for Kennedy's unilateral termination of atmospheric testing?

  A. The revelation that his defense advisors wanted additional atmospheric tests to determine the impact of nuclear weapons on neighboring regions

  B. The revelation that his defense advisors opposed the termination of testing, arguing that it would be taken as a sign of weakness

  C. A report that the Soviets were preparing to announce a unilateral termination of their strategic bomber production

  D. A finding that Kennedy was initially opposed to the idea of a cessation of atmospheric testing

GO ON TO THE NEXT PAGE.

27. President Kennedy's suggestion to Americans to reexamine their attitudes toward the cold war (lines 30-33) suggests that before his speech, the prevalent attitude of Americans toward the cold war was:

A. inflexible: the Soviets were a dangerous, implacable enemy
B. ambivalent: most people did not expect the cold war to have a direct effect on their lives
C. resentful: the American government was spending too much on nuclear weapons
D. smug: the American military was far superior to that of the Soviets

28. Implicit in the passage is the idea that:

A. because of his assassination, President Kennedy never followed through on his plans.
B. unilateral disarmament is superior to bilateral disarmament.
C. despite the superiority of the American strategic military forces, a peace with the Communists was more desirable than a "hot war" with them.
D. if the cold war could be prolonged for long enough without becoming "hot," the superior American economy would eventually cause the Soviet Union to collapse.

29. If President Kennedy desired to make another unilateral "psychological gesture," which of the following actions would have qualified?

A. asking the Soviets to attend a conference on the peaceful uses of outer space
B. announcing a program to develop an anti-ballistic missile
C. dropping leaflets on Cuba that support a counter-revolution
D. extending formal recognition to a Communist delegation already recognized by the United Nations

30. In line 39, the termination of atmospheric testing is referred to as "not a unilateral arms limitation step." Which of the following would have qualified as a unilateral arms limitation step?

A. removing obsolete submarines from the fleet
B. discontinuing the development of new strategic bombers
C. offering to cut the number of American nuclear missiles by 50% if the Soviets did likewise
D. calling on the world to follow America's lead in halting atmospheric testing

---

GO ON TO THE NEXT PAGE.

Copyright © 2001 EXAMKRACKERS, Inc.

The idea that it was within the power of the visual arts to change the moral dimension of life reached its peak between the death of Monroe and that of Lincoln. One sees it in full bloom in the weekly editorials in *The Crayon*, New York's main art magazine in the 1850s. It was the voice of the American artist's profession and, as such, held strong views on artists' character and conduct. As the editor bluntly put it in 1855, "The enjoyment of beauty is dependent on, and in ratio with, the moral excellence of the individual. We have assumed that Art is an elevating power, that is has *in itself* a spirit of morality." The first form of the American artist as culture-hero, then, is a preacher. He raised art from being mere craft by moral utterance. God was the supreme artist; they imitated His work, the "Book of Nature." They divided the light and calmed the waters—especially if they were Boston Luminists. They were a counterweight to American materialism.

What was art for?, the *Crayon* asked, in what is called "this hard, angular and groveling age," the 1850s [sic]. Why, it was to show the artist as "a reformer, a philanthropist, full of hope and reverence and love." And if he slipped, he fell a long way, like Lucifer. "If the reverence of men is to be given to Art," warned another editorial, "especial care must be taken that it is not…offered in foul and unseemly vessels. We judge religion by the character of those who represent and embody it…"

Under the influence of the Romantic movement, the desire for art as religion changed; it was gradually supplanted by a taste for the Romantic sublime, still morally instructive, but more indefinite and secular. The Hudson River painters created their images of American nature as God's fingerprint; Frederick Church and Albert Bierstadt made immense landscapes that gave Americans all the traits of Romantic art— size, virtuosity, surrender to prodigy and spectacle— except for one: its anxiety. The American wilderness, in their hand, never makes you feel insecure. It is Eden; its God is an American God whose gospel is Manifest Destiny. It is not the world of Turner or Géricault, with its intimations of disaster and death. Nor is it the field of experience that some American *writing* had claimed—Melville's sense of the catastrophic, or Poe's morbid self-enclosure. It is pious, public, and full of uplift.

No wonder it was so popular with the growing American art audience in the 1870s and 1880s. For this audience expected art to grant it relief from the dark side of life. It didn't like either Romantic anguish or realism. There is a strange absence from American painting at this time, like the dog that didn't bark in the night. It is the refusal to deal in any explicit way with the immense social trauma of the Civil War. American art, apart from illustration, hardly mentions the war at all. The sense of pity, fratricidal horror and social waste that pervades the writing of the time, like Walt Whitman, and is still surfacing thirty years later in Stephen Crane's *Red Badge of Courage,* is only to be *seen* in arranged battlefield photographs like those of Mathew Brady—never in painting. This is a curious outcome, particularly if you believe, as I do, that the best strand in 19th-century American art is not so much the Romantic-nationalist one of Bierstadt and Church, but the line of virile, empirical sight that runs from Audubon through Eakins and Homer.

31. According to the passage, which of the following most likely describes the change in 19th century American painting during the Romantic movement?

 A. American painting lost its religious overtones.
 B. Overt religious depiction gave way to reverent innuendo.
 C. Tense and exciting images replaced scenes of silent worship.
 D. Paintings of loving couples began to appear more often than those of devout religious characters.

32. According to the passage, which of the following might be found in a Romantic painting but not in a 19th century American painting?

 A. A beautiful mountain range with snow covered peaks.
 B. A small, lone church nestled in the pine trees of a large valley.
 C. A proud American Indian surveying the open plains.
 D. Terrified townspeople fleeing for cover from ominous storm clouds encroaching upon their small town.

GO ON TO THE NEXT PAGE.

33. According to the passage, the American Civil War was portrayed mainly in:

    I. American painting
    II. Romantic painting
    III. Novels
    IV. Photography

    A. II only
    B. II and III only
    C. I and IV only
    D. III and IV only

34. The author would probably consider which of the following to be most similar in spirit to American painting of the 1870s and 1880s?

    A. European Romantic painting of the same period
    B. Herman Melville's *Moby Dick*
    C. American musicals of the 1950's
    D. Journalistic photographs of the Vietnam War

35. According to the passage, in which of the following ways did American art of the 1870s differ from that of the 1850s?

    I. Art in the 1870s was more realistic.
    II. Art in the 1870s is more depressing.
    III. Art in the 1870s is not meant to be inspiring.

    A. I only
    B. III only
    C. I and II only
    D. None of these

36. From the passage, it can be inferred that most Americans living in the 1870s:

    A. longed for the "good old days" of the 1850s.
    B. felt that they lived in a golden age of happiness and plenty.
    C. had abandoned religion.
    D. wanted art to distract them from real life.

37. According to the passage, which of the following was responsible for the shift in art between the 1850s and the 1870s?

    A. The Civil War
    B. The Romantic movement
    C. The development of photography
    D. The influence of literature

38. Which of the following were characteristics of Romantic art?

    I. Concentration on the personal and individual as opposed to the grand and heroic
    II. A high degree of technical skill
    III. A cheerful, upbeat feel

    A. I only
    B. II only
    C. I and III only
    D. I, II, and III

GO ON TO THE NEXT PAGE.

Passage III (Questions 39-46)

Much of the western and especially the American press tends to take a *monolinear* approach to the "transition" of Russia and the other former Communist states, according to which they are all on one "path" to
5 "democracy and the free market." They may proceed at different speeds, stop, or even go backward, but the assumption is that the ultimate goal is one and indivisible, and that you can take only one monorail route to get there.

10 The most sophisticated contemporary version of this is, of course, Francis Fukuyama's "end of history" thesis. In the American media, a shallow, bland version of Fukuyama's thought is so omnipresent that it is rarely noticed, let alone analyzed or criticized. A
15 classic, and typical, example appeared in a 1996 Washington Post article. The subject was the Armenians, but exactly the same formula has been used to describe all the former Communist countries that have undergone "reform." The correspondent wrote that "after Soviet
20 rule and war with Azerbaijan, [Armenians] are getting back on the path of free markets and democracy, albeit with growing pains."

Leaving aside the truly horrible mixed metaphor— after all, what do you do if you suffer growing pains
25 while on a path? Retire behind a tree?—this sentence in its short life succeeds in promiscuously coupling with no fewer than four ideological assumptions, all of doubtful character.

The first is the religious imagery bound up with the
30 metaphor of a "path," evocative of spiritual quests, pilgrimages, and the pursuit of various species of Grail. Except for rare revolutionary moments, the use of religious metaphors for political processes is usually a mistake. Everywhere and most of the time, the
35 principal business of politics is politics: it is the process by which people try to acquire and keep power, the wealth that comes from power, or the power to protect wealth. We all know this instinctively when we look at our own politicians; but too often, when reporting on
40 other countries, we assume that their political processes are somehow much more driven by ideological quests.

Second, reinforcing the religious metaphor, with its implications of the nobility of the aim, is the organic metaphor of "growing pains," which implies an
45 inevitable and scientifically determined process by which a life, unless artificially cut short, develops according to certain fixed rules toward an inevitable end. States and nations, while they may develop in some sense organically, do not do so after the fashion
50 of individual organisms. Rather, they are like complex ecosystems in which if one element changes, it unpredictably influences the rest until in the end the whole system has been transformed.

Third, there is the assumption that before this organic
55 process was interrupted by Soviet rule, Armenia and other nations in the region were proceeding along this path to "democracy and the free market." This was true of Estonia and Latvia, and possibly of Georgia; but in the case of Armenia and other areas, their history before
60 the Soviet annexation, and the ideology of their leading nationalist parties, allows no such confidence.

Finally, there is the monolithic attitude that colors the entire passage. It speaks of the path to democracy (evidently viewed as taking a single form, already fixed
65 and fully understood) and the free market. But the way capitalist economies work and are influenced by states differs immensely from country to country; the paths by which countries have developed capitalism are highly varied, and for every truly "free" electoral system there
70 is another that is rigged, bought, managed, or shaped according to local patterns and traditions. It is also true of course that for every fully successful capitalist state there are two or three where for many decades progress has proved halting and ambiguous, especially as far as
75 the mass of the population is concerned. There is nothing "abnormal" in the world today about the states of Egypt, Mexico, and Pakistan. (Ironically, as the Post article on Armenia appeared, the Armenian government was itself following a "normal" pattern by preparing to
80 rig an election and crack down on the opposition.)

Analysis based on the monolinear view of development is mistaken with regard to most countries in the world. When applied to Russia, it can become actively dangerous, because it can so easily tie in with
85 prejudices about the "perennial" Russian character. If there is only one path forward, then this logically means that there is only one path back: either the development of a pro-Western, free-market democracy, or a reversion to "dictatorship and aggressive external
90 policies."

And when the Western belief in a single road to democracy becomes mixed up with the ideological belief that "democracies do not go to war with each other," whereas dictatorships are naturally prone to
95 aggression, then the layers of mystification become almost impenetrable.

GO ON TO THE NEXT PAGE.

39. The main point as expressed by the author is:

   A. Russia is a special case when it comes to development of democracy.
   B. Political development is a unique process in each country, and the result is not necessarily a democracy.
   C. The final stage of political development in any country is democracy.
   D. The road to democracy is rarely straight and smooth.

40. According to the passage, Fukiyama's "end of history" thesis most likely describes:

   A. the natural progression of systems of government in a single country.
   B. Russia's struggle to become a democratic nation.
   C. four common ideological errors concerning the political development of nations.
   D. free market and democracy in post-Soviet Armenia.

41. The author believes that the *monolinear* view is actively dangerous when applied to Russia because:

   A. any lateral move by Russia will derail its efforts toward a democracy.
   B. Russia will be unable to circumvent obstacles and will be forced to crash through them.
   C. governments may act on the assumption that if Russia fails to develop its democracy in a similar fashion to the U.S., then Russia must be returning to communism.
   D. the Russian character is deeply imbedded, and Russians may be hostile to the expectations of foreigners.

42. Which of the following best represents the author's attitude toward western ideas concerning democracy?

   A. exaggerated incredulity
   B. sincere fascination
   C. arrogant disregard
   D. anxiously critical

43. The author probably views the Mexican government as:

   A. a fully successful capitalist state.
   B. a truly free electoral system.
   C. rigged, bought, managed, or shaped according to local traditions.
   D. being on the path toward democracy.

44. Suppose a U.S. congressman cites the first amendment to defend the right of tobacco companies to advertise on television. The author of the passage would most likely believe that the politician:

   A. was sincerely concerned that the constitution might be violated.
   B. used tobacco himself.
   C. had been bribed.
   D. was more concerned with protecting the wealth of the tobacco companies than with defending the constitution.

45. According to the author, if not for Soviet intervention, Armenia today would:

   A. be a democracy.
   B. be on a similar path to democracy as that taken by the U.S.
   C. be on a path to democracy, but probably different to the one taken by the U.S.
   D. probably not be a democracy.

46. The author most likely believes that wars are caused by:

   A. ideological differences in governments.
   B. political entities struggling to protect or increase their wealth.
   C. philosophical differences between the people of the warring nations.
   D. international incidents resulting in misunderstandings between nations.

STOP. IF YOU FINISH BEFORE TIME IS CALLED, CHECK YOUR WORK. YOU MAY GO BACK TO ANY QUESTION IN THIS TEST BOOKLET.

STOP.

30-minute
In-class Exam
for Lecture 3

Passage I (Questions 47-53)

In November of 1918 an armistice ended what was then called the Great War, but that armistice could not halt the even greater ravages of an influenza virus. In four years the armies of Europe killed more than 8 million soldiers and nearly as many civilians while barely moving their front lines. In the course of a single year, beginning in the spring of 1918, the virus managed to invade the entire world and kill more than 20 million of its inhabitants. No region was spared as the contagion, following trade routes and shipping lines, swept across Africa, Asia, Europe, North America, and the South Pacific. The origins of the virus and the reasons for its unusual virulence are still unknown.

No one imagined, then or now, that the killer flu was a deliberate act of war. Nonetheless, the demonstrated potential impressed the statesmen of the era. When the Geneva Protocol was issued in 1925 to ban the use of the poison gas that had evoked special revulsion on the World War I battlefields, the provision was extended to include bacteriological agents as well. The protocol affirmed that weapons of both types were "justly condemned by the general opinion of the civilized world."

More than 70 years later, revulsion persists and the Geneva Protocol has been strengthened, but the sense of threat of biological warfare has intensified. It is widely recognized that, as potential instruments of destruction, biological agents are inexpensive, readily accessible, and unusually dangerous. Of the thousands of pathogens that prey upon human beings, a few are now known to have the potential for causing truly massive devastation, with mortality levels conceivably exceeding what chemical or even nuclear weapons could produce. Nature provides the prototypes without requiring any design bureau or manufacturing facility. Medical science provides increasingly useful information, which by its very nature is conveyed in open literature. A small home-brewery is all that would be required to produce a potent threat of major pro-portions. At least 17 countries are suspected of conducting biological weapons research—including several, such as Iran and Iraq, that are especially hostile to the United States.

It is a considerable comfort and undoubtedly a key to our survival that, so far, the main lines of defense against this threat have not depended on explicit policies or organized efforts. In the long course of evolution, the human body has developed physical barriers and a biochemical immune system whose sophistication and effectiveness exceed anything we could design or as yet even fully understand. But evolution is a sword that cuts both ways: New diseases emerge, while old diseases mutate and adapt. Throughout history, there have been epidemics during which human immunity has broken down on an epic scale.... As we enter the twenty-first century, changing conditions have enhanced the potential for widespread contagion. The rapid growth rate of the total world population, the unprecedented freedom of movement across international borders, and scientific advances that expand the capability for the deliberate manipulation of pathogens are all cause for worry that the problem might be greater in the future than it has ever been in the past. The threat of infectious pathogens is not just an issue of public health, but a fundamental security problem for the species as a whole.

In recent years, this realization has begun to seep into international security deliberations.... [T]he United States has strengthened legal authority to preempt terrorist threats, has established more extensive regulations for handling hazardous biological agents, and has created for the first time special military units continuously prepared to respond to domestic incidents. Internationally, negotiations are under way to strengthen the Biological and Toxin Weapons Convention (BWC).... But these efforts are merely tentative first steps toward dealing with a problem that vitally affects the entire human population. Ultimately the world's military, medical, and business establishments will have to work together to an unprecedented degree if the international community is to succeed in containing the threat of biological weapons.

47. The central thesis of the passage is that:

A. biological weapons should be outlawed for use in war.

B. biological weapons are capable of greater destruction than chemical or nuclear weapons.

C. due to the accessibility and lethal potency of biological weapons, a coordinated international effort is required to prevent their use.

D. biological weapons are nothing more than the newest technology in a long line of weapons of mass destruction.

48. When the author says "evolution is a sword that cuts both ways," (line 53) he is most likely referring to:

A. the advance of technology and the decline of the natural defenses of the human body.
B. the human body's ability to fight disease and a pathogen's ability to overcome the body's defenses.
C. progressive and regressive evolution.
D. the loss of immunity against certain pathogens due to the evolution of the human body.

49. The author implies that which of the following has acted as a deterrent to the spread of nuclear weapons among countries hostile to the U.S.?

A. the threat of government sanctions
B. the advanced technology required to assemble nuclear weapons
C. U.S. military presence in areas where a threat may exist
D. condemnation by the civilized world

50. The *main lines of defense* (line 46) most likely refers to:

A. modern medicine.
B. special military units designed to respond to biological hazards.
C. international acts such as the Geneva Protocol.
D. the human immune system.

51. Which of the following would the author most likely view as posing the greatest danger to students at a high school in the U.S.?

A. a hand gun shop located near the high school
B. a student coming to school while sick with the flu
C. instructions on the internet explaining how to manufacture pipe bombs from materials found in the home
D. a fire

52. According to the passage, why haven't biological weapons been a threat to international security until now?

A. The threat from more potent weapons, such as nuclear explosives, has only recently been contained.
B. The technology required to create a pathogen capable of overcoming the human immune system was achieved this century.
C. Global internet has provided access to information previously unavailable to the public.
D. Until now, no country could overcome U.S. hegemony.

53. The influenza virus is mentioned as an example of:

A. an effective biological weapon used in the past.
B. the devastative potential inherent in biological weapons.
C. one possible biological weapon that may be used in the future.
D. how the losing side of a war may exact revenge for an unjust treaty using biological weapons.

_____

GO ON TO THE NEXT PAGE.

Passage II (Questions 54-61)

In the 1930s widespread recession became world depression only after countries retreated behind tariff walls and trade collapsed. Today the world economy wobbles and teeters, but most governments vow that they have learnt their lesson. Perhaps they have. Even so, it is reassuring that international trade rules make a return to protection harder and more expensive than it was in the 1930s:

Do not bank on it. For there is a big hole in those multilateral rules. Countries can slap duties on cheap imports that they judge are being *dumped* in their markets. And—surprise, surprise—there has recently been a surge in anti-dumping cases around the world, as companies such as America's steel makers feel the pinch of slowing growth and rising imports from crisis-hit economies.

Anti-dumping is a particularly pernicious form of *protection*, because it lurks beneath a veneer of respectability. Its apologists assert not merely that foreigners are stealing jobs at home—the usual protectionist line—but that they are doing so unfairly by selling their wares on the cheap, perhaps in the hope of driving domestic competitors out of business. Anti-dumpers claim to target only such cheats; and, moreover, to use objective calculations of what they ought to charge, making proper allowance for profit. Duties are imposed only to bring prices back into line with what they should be; if victims squeal, they can raise their prices instead.

Yet the practice is very different from the theory. Dumping calculations are a sham. Foreigners are almost always found at fault. Huge duties are imposed and rarely removed, even when conditions change. Worse still are the hidden costs of anti-dumping. A government that threatens any foreign firm offering the keenest prices is merely encouraging it and others to raise prices and cut sales. In effect, companies are being urged to collude at consumers' expense.

But surely anti-dumping measures may be justified if foreigners are guilty of *predatory pricing*? Not usually. Genuine predatory pricing is extremely rare, because it relies on the unlikely ability of a single producer to dominate a world market. In any case, consumers gain from lower prices; so do companies that can buy their supplies more cheaply abroad—General Motors, for example, in the case of steel. And even in the very few cases where foreigners might drive domestic producers out of business and raise prices once they corner the market, anti-dumping is the wrong response.

A better answer would be to invite national antitrust authorities, who look into predatory pricing by domestic firms, to deal with foreigners too. That is how this matter is dealt with between Australia and New Zealand. A further improvement would be to write antitrust rules into world trade law. Competition policy may be on the agenda for next year's trade summit in Washington, DC, which could launch a new round of trade talks. Its remit could easily be widened to cover anti-dumping as well as other competition issues.

As of now, however, such a change looks unlikely. America seems wedded to anti-dumping, as does the European Commission. Both are encouraging hard-pressed domestic producers to seek protection, sometimes by filing repeat cases, often starting one up immediately after another has been turned down. Now other countries are retaliating with anti-dumping suits of their own against American and European firms. As the cases multiply, a mockery is made of multilateral efforts to fend off protection. In short, the echoes of the 1930s may yet reverberate. It is time for the world to dump anti-dumping.

54. Which of the following statements best summarizes the main idea of the passage?

A. International trade rules against protectionism protect the world economy from a second depression.

B. Environmental protectionists risk plunging the world economy into a recession with anti-dumping laws.

C. Certain international laws which are meant to protect domestic companies against unfair trade practices of foreign competitors are bad for the global economy and should be expunged.

D. Anti-dumping laws are misused by American and European companies.

55. The author of this passage would probably give his *greatest* support to which of the following?

A. Duties imposed by the U.S. congress on the goods of foreign companies engaging in predatory pricing practices

B. Abolition of all international trade laws

C. Legalization of international *predatory pricing* practices

D. International efforts other than dumping laws that prevent the domination of any market by one company

GO ON TO THE NEXT PAGE.

56. Which of the following are mentioned in the passage as exacerbating the problems created by anti-dumping laws?

    I. Slow domestic growth
    II. Foreigners guilty of predatory pricing
   III. Weakened foreign economies

    A. II only
    B. I and II only
    C. I and III only
    D. I, II, and III

57. Based on the passage, which of the following is NOT true concerning *predatory pricing*?

    A. It always involves a foreign company.
    B. One company must have a controlling share of the market.
    C. Prices are unjustly lowered to gain market share.
    D. It is against international trade rules.

58. The author most likely believes that the depression of the 1930s was the result of:

    A. protectionist policies throughout the world.
    B. predatory pricing.
    C. anti-dumping laws.
    D. international antitrust legislation.

59. The author's attitude toward the *protectionist* point of view can best be described as:

    A. contemptuous
    B. respectful disagreement
    C. supportive
    D. apathetic

60. *Dumping calculations* (line 31) most likely refer to:

    A. estimates of the number of foreign companies practicing dumping.
    B. a specific plan to lower the prices of imports.
    C. intentional persecution of importers.
    D. mathematical formulas used by the court to identify acts of predatory pricing.

61. Which of the following assertions does the author support with evidence, explanation, or examples?

    I. Anti-dumping laws have hidden costs
    II. Tariffs made a major contribution to the 1930s depression.
   III. Some companies benefit from predatory pricing.

    A. I only
    B. I and II only
    C. I and III only
    D. I, II, and III

GO ON TO THE NEXT PAGE.

From the porch where I am slumped, exhausted by the heat, I stare in astonishment at a man walking up the forest trail from the beach, snorkel dangling from one hand. I have just arrived at Dugong Creek, a remote corner of Little Andaman Island in the Bay of Bengal, to meet the Onges, a group of hunter-gatherers believed to be descended from Asia's first humans. I hadn't expected to find other visitors.

"You know there are crocodiles," I say, indicating his snorkel.

"A hazard of the trade," he grins. Himansu S. Das of the Salim Ali Center for Ornithology and Natural History in Coimbatore, India, is a sea-grass ecologist. Because dugongs, Old World relatives of the manatee, feed on underwater greenery, he had guessed that Dugong Creek would have beds of sea grass nearby. The animals themselves, though, were likely to be long gone. Once seen in the hundreds or even thousands along the tropical coasts of Africa and Asia, these sea elephants are all but extinct in most of their range and occur in reasonable numbers only in Australia. In five years of exploration, Das has gathered evidence of at most 40 dugongs throughout the Andaman and Nicobar archipelago. To his surprise, he has just learned from the Onges that a family of four still lives in Dugong Creek, down one since their hunt of two weeks ago.

The grass beds nourish not only these rare mammals but also marine turtles and a variety of fish and shellfish. With the help of a grant from UNESCO, Das is estimating the impact of humans on the ecology. In fact, it is the local peoples who point him to the beds, more predictably than do the satellite images on which he initially relied.

The next afternoon, under a blistering sun, we set out for an Onge camp a kilometer or so along the shore. At one point we have to ford a creek. Halfway across, in chest-deep water and with my sandals held aloft in one hand, it strikes me.

"Crocodiles?" I ask.

"Just keep walking," he replies. I do. Saltwater crocodiles are the most ferocious of them all, and I've seen their tracks on the beach.

The Onges, we discover; have not seen a dugong but have harpooned two turtles. One is being cooked, and the other is secured at the end of a long rope stretched into the sea. When Koira, an Onge man, pulls on the leash, a head sticks anxiously out of the water as the animal looks to see where it is being drawn. It is an endangered green sea turtle, small, about 15 kilograms.

Neither of us begrudges the Onges their meal. They have lived on Little Andaman for millennia with no harm to its biodiversity and now, because of pressure from recent settlers, will probably vanish long before the turtles. The main threat to the sea-grass beds and to the creatures that depend on them is the silt that muddies the water as the dense tropical forest is cut down: the marine plants die of darkness. Overexploitation of fish, shellfish and other marine species by immigrants from mainland India and by fishers from as far away as Thailand is another pressing problem.

As the grass patches shrink, the dugongs become confined to ever smaller regions that are also the local fishing grounds. Some fishers set their nets around the beds to catch predators, such as sharks, that come to feed on smaller fish, but the nets entangle turtles as well as an occasional dugong. Das will be recommending to the Indian authorities that some sea-grass beds be protected as sanctuaries. But as we return—the tide has gone out, mercifully leaving the creek just knee-deep— I realize with sadness that it's already too late for the Andaman dugong.

62. Which of the following statements best summarizes the main idea of the passage?

   A. The pressures of modern civilization are forcing primitive societies to hunt endangered species like the dugong to extinction.
   B. The destruction of natural habitat has doomed the dugong and others in Dugong Creek to extinction.
   C. The Andaman dugong can only be saved if we act now.
   D. Dugongs and other rare animals are nourished by the vanishing grass beds of Dugong creek.

63. Which of the following is the most likely explanation for the destruction of the tropical forest around Dugong Creek?

   A. The Onges slash and burn land to cultivate crops.
   B. Large lumber corporations exploit the land.
   C. The expansion of a nearby city.
   D. Island residents other than the Onges clearing land.

64. The tone of the author is best characterized as one of:

   A. cautious optimism.
   B. ominous foreboding.
   C. doleful acceptance.
   D. controlled rage.

GO ON TO THE NEXT PAGE.

65. Which of the following explains why the author is thankful that the creek is *only knee-deep* (line 69)?

A. He fears an attack by a saltwater crocodile.
B. He is probably a poor swimmer.
C. He is weary and tired, and doesn't wish to be wet.
D. The dugong are safer in the shallow water.

66. Which of the following might the author propose as the most effective method to save the dugongs?

A. Protect many sea-grass beds as sanctuaries.
B. Prevent the Onges from hunting dugongs.
C. Halt deforestation near dugong habitats.
D. Pass a law barring net fishing around the sea-grass beds.

67. In line 32, the author probably mentions *satellite images* in order to demonstrate:

A. man's complete control of his environment.
B. man's inability to dominate nature.
C. the extreme accuracy of scientific research.
D. the cold, barren future of man without nature.

68. Which of the following is implied in the passage?

A. It is too late to save dugongs from world extinction.
B. Africa currently has the largest dugong populations.
C. Dugong Creek dugongs need clear water to thrive.
D. Saltwater crocodiles eat dugongs.

69. With which of the following would the author most likely agree?

A. Advanced technology may be mankind's last hope to preserve the environment.
B. Mankind will never dominate nature, but may destroy nature in the attempt.
C. Nature is resilient enough to rebound from any blow.
D. All technology is bad.

STOP. IF YOU FINISH BEFORE TIME IS CALLED, CHECK YOUR WORK. YOU MAY GO BACK TO ANY QUESTION IN THIS TEST BOOKLET.

STOP.

Answers to 30
minute exams:

Lecture 1

1. C
2. D
3. C
4. A
5. B
6. A
7. D
8. D
9. D
10. A
11. C
12. B
13. A
14. C
15. D
16. B
17. D
18. C
19. B
20. C
21. C
22. C
23. D

Lecture 2

24. C
25. D
26. A
27. A
28. C
29. D
30. B
31. B
32. D
33. D
34. C
35. D
36. D
37. B
38. B
39. B
40. A
41. C

42. A
43. C
44. D
45. D
46. B

Lecture 3

47. C
48. B
49. B
50. D
51. C
52. B
53. B
54. C
55. D
56. C
57. A
58. A
59. A
60. D
61. C
62. B
63. D
64. C
65. A
66. C
67. B
68. C
69. B

Homework

1. A
2. C
3. A
4. A
5. D
6. D
7. C

Stand Alones

1. B
2. A
3. B
4. B
5. A
6. D
7. A
8. B
9. D
10. B
11. D
12. D
13. A
14. D
15. A
16. C
17. D
18. C
19. C
20. A
21. B
22. B
23. A

Reading Comprehension	
Raw Score	**Estimated Scaled Score**
23	13-15
22	12
20-21	11
19	10
17-18	9
16	8
15	7
12-14	6
11	5
10	4

About the Author

Jonathan Orsay is uniquely qualified to write an MCAT preparation book. He graduated on the Dean's list with a B.A. in History from Columbia University. While considering medical school, he sat for the real MCAT three times from 1989 to 1996. He scored in the 90 percentiles on all sections before becoming an MCAT instructor. He has lectured in MCAT test preparation for thousands of hours and across the country for every MCAT administration since August 1994. He has taught premeds from such prestigious Universities as Harvard and Columbia. He was the editor of one of the best selling MCAT prep books in 1996 and again in 1997. Orsay is currently the Director of MCAT for Examkrackers. He has written and published the following books and audio products in MCAT preparation: "Examkrackers MCAT Physics"; "Examkrackers MCAT Chemistry"; "Examkrackers MCAT Organic Chemistry"; "Examkrackers MCAT Biology"; "Examkrackers MCAT Verbal Reasoning & Math"; "Examkrackers 1001 questions in MCAT Physics", "Examkrackers MCAT Audio Osmosis with Jordan and Jon".

An Unedited Student Review of This Book

The following review of this book was written by Teri R---. from New York. Teri scored a 43 out of 45 possible points on the MCAT. She is currently attending UCSF medical school, one of the most selective medical schools in the country.

The Examkrackers MCAT books are the best MCAT prep materials I've seen-and I looked at many before deciding. The worst part about studying for the MCAT is figuring out what you need to cover and getting the material organized. These books do all that for you so that you can spend your time learning. The books are well and carefully written, with great diagrams and really useful mnemonic tricks, so you don't waste time trying to figure out what the book is saying. They are concise enough that you can get through all of the subjects without cramming unnecessary details, and they really give you a strategy for the exam. The study questions in each section cover all the important concepts, and let you check your learning after each section. Alternating between reading and answering questions in MCAT format really helps make the material stick, and means there are no surprises on the day of the exam-the exam format seems really familiar and this helps enormously with the anxiety. Basically, these books make it clear what you need to do to be completely prepared for the MCAT and deliver it to you in a straightforward and easy-to-follow form. The mass of material you could study is overwhelming, so I decided to trust these books--I used nothing but the Examkrackers books in all subjects and got a 13-15 on Verbal, a 14 on Physical Sciences, and a 14 on Biological Sciences. Thanks to Jonathan Orsay and Examkrackers, I was admitted to all of my top-choice schools (Columbia, Cornell, Stanford, and UCSF). I will always be grateful. I could not recommend the Examkrackers books more strongly. Please contact me if you have any questions.

Sincerely,
Teri R----

About the Author

Jonathan Orsay is uniquely qualified to write an MCAT preparation book. He graduated on the Dean's list with a B.A. in History from Columbia University. While considering medical school, he sat for the real MCAT three times from 1989 to 1996. He scored in the 90 percentiles on all sections before becoming an MCAT instructor. He has lectured in MCAT test preparation for thousands of hours and across the country for every MCAT administration since August 1994. He has taught premeds from such prestigious Universities as Harvard and Columbia. He was the editor of one of the best selling MCAT prep books in 1996 and again in 1997. Orsay is currently the Director of MCAT for Examkrackers. He has written and published the following books and audio products in MCAT preparation: "Examkrackers MCAT Physics"; "Examkrackers MCAT Chemistry"; "Examkrackers MCAT Organic Chemistry"; "Examkrackers MCAT Biology"; "Examkrackers MCAT Verbal Reasoning & Math"; "Examkrackers 1001 questions in MCAT Physics", "Examkrackers MCAT Audio Osmosis with Jordan and Jon".

An Unedited Student Review of This Book

The following review of this book was written by Teri R---. from New York. Teri scored a 43 out of 45 possible points on the MCAT. She is currently attending UCSF medical school, one of the most selective medical schools in the country.

The Examkrackers MCAT books are the best MCAT prep materials I've seen-and I looked at many before deciding. The worst part about studying for the MCAT is figuring out what you need to cover and getting the material organized. These books do all that for you so that you can spend your time learning. The books are well and carefully written, with great diagrams and really useful mnemonic tricks, so you don't waste time trying to figure out what the book is saying. They are concise enough that you can get through all of the subjects without cramming unnecessary details, and they really give you a strategy for the exam. The study questions in each section cover all the important concepts, and let you check your learning after each section. Alternating between reading and answering questions in MCAT format really helps make the material stick, and means there are no surprises on the day of the exam-the exam format seems really familiar and this helps enormously with the anxiety. Basically, these books make it clear what you need to do to be completely prepared for the MCAT and deliver it to you in a straightforward and easy-to-follow form. The mass of material you could study is overwhelming, so I decided to trust these books--I used nothing but the Examkrackers books in all subjects and got a 13-15 on Verbal, a 14 on Physical Sciences, and a 14 on Biological Sciences. Thanks to Jonathan Orsay and Examkrackers, I was admitted to all of my top-choice schools (Columbia, Cornell, Stanford, and UCSF). I will always be grateful. I could not recommend the Examkrackers books more strongly. Please contact me if you have any questions.

Sincerely,
Teri R----